OPCS Surveys of Psychiatric Morbidity in Great Britain

Report 1

The prevalence of psychiatric morbidity among adults living in private households

Howard Meltzer

Baljit Gill

Mark Petticrew

Kerstin Hinds

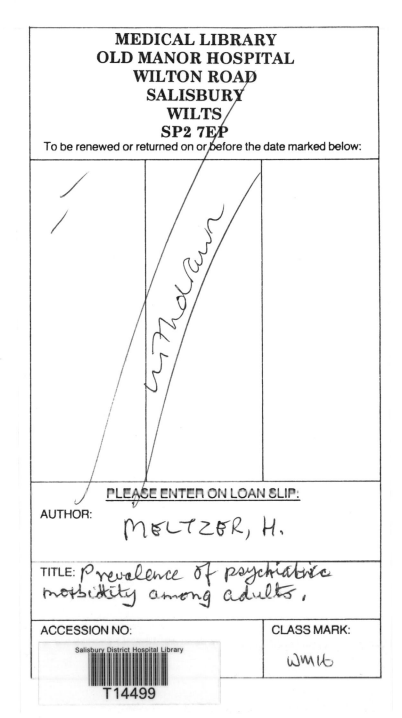

London: HMSO

ISBN 0 11 691627 3

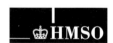

Published by HMSO and available from:

HMSO Publications Centre
(Mail, fax and telephone orders only)
PO Box 276, London, SW8 5DT
Telephone orders 0171 873 9090
General enquiries 0171 873 0011
(queuing system in operation for both numbers)
Fax orders 0171 873 8200

HMSO Bookshops
49 High Holborn, London, WC1V 6HB
(counter service only)
0171 873 0011 Fax 0171 831 1326
68–69 Bull Street, Birmingham B4 6AD
0121 236 9696 Fax 0121 236 9699
33 Wine Street, Bristol, BS1 2BQ
0117 9264306 Fax 0117 9294515
9-21 Princess Street, Manchester, M60 8AS
0161 834 7201 Fax 0161 833 0634
16 Arthur Street, Belfast, BT1 4GD
01232 238451 Fax 01232 235401
71 Lothian Road, Edinburgh, EH3 9AZ
0131 228 4181 Fax 0131 229 2734
The HMSO Oriel Bookshop
The Friary, Cardiff CF1 4AA
01222 395548 Fax 01222 384347

HMSO's Accredited Agents
(see Yellow Pages)

and through good booksellers

Authors' acknowledgements

We would like to thank everybody who contributed to the survey and the production of this Report. We were supported by our specialist colleagues in OPCS who carried out the sampling, fieldwork, coding and editing stages.

Great thanks are due to the interviewers who worked on the survey and to the Registrars of Psychiatry who conducted the SCAN interviews.

The project was steered by a group comprising the following, to whom thanks are due for assistance and specialist advice at various stages of the survey:

Department of Health:
Dr Rachel Jenkins (chair)
Dr Elaine Gadd
Ms Val Roberts
Mr Alan Madge

Psychiatric epidemiologists:
Dr Paul Bebbington
Dr Terry Brugha
Dr Glyn Lewis
Dr Mike Farrell
Dr Jacquie de Alarcon

Office of Population Censuses and Surveys:
Ms Jil Matheson
Dr Howard Meltzer
Ms Baljit Gill
Dr Mark Petticrew
Ms Kerstin Hinds

We would also like to acknowledge Dr Scott Weich of the Institute of Psychiatry for his work on the diagnostic guidelines for the CIS-R.

Most importantly, we would like to thank all the participants in the survey for their time and co-operation

Contents

List of tables

Chapter 6: Prevalence of psychiatric disorders

List of figures

Notes

Tables showing percentages

The row or column percentages may add to 99% or 101% because of rounding.

The varying positions of the percentage signs and bases in the tables denote the presentation of different types of information. Where there is a percentage sign at the head of a column and the base at the foot, the whole distribution is presented and the individual percentages add to between 99% and 101%. Where there is no percentage sign in the table and a note above the figures, the figures refer to the proportion of people who had the attribute being discussed, and the complimentary proportion, to add to 100%, is not shown in the table.

Standard errors are shown in brackets beside percentages in the tables.

The following conventions have been used within tables showing percentages:
-      no cases
- 0   values less than 0.5%

Tables showing odds ratios

In the analysis for this Report, odds ratios were calculated when logistic regression was carried out. The logistic regression identified, from a range of variables, those which were independently related to specific symptoms/disorders. Odds ratios (ORs) were produced only for those variables where a significant relationship was identified. More information about the logistic regression model used is included in Appendix D.

In the tables showing ORs, asterisks are used to denote the level of statistical significance for differences between categories. For each variable a reference group was selected (OR=1.00) and the other groups were compared with this group. The way in which reference groups were selected and the impact of this on analysis is explained in Appendix D.

Significant differences

The bases for some sub-groups presented in the tables were small such that the standard errors around estimates for these groups are biased. Confidence intervals which take account of these biased standard errors were calculated and, although they are not presented in the tables, they were used in testing for statistically significant differences. Statistical significance is explained in Appendix D of this Report.

Prevalence of neurotic disorders

This Report was preceded by a Bulletin (published in December 1994)[1] which presented preliminary findings of the survey. There are minor differences in the figures given for the prevalence of neurotic disorders in the Bulletin and this Report; data presented in this Report should be used in place of those in the Bulletin.

[1] Meltzer, H., Gill, B., and Petticrew, M., (1994) *OPCS Surveys of Psychiatric Morbidity in Great Britain, Bulletin No.1: The prevalence of psychiatric morbidity among adults aged 16-64, living in private households, in Great Britain*, OPCS, London

Summary

The OPCS Surveys of psychiatric morbidity in Great Britain were commissioned by the Department of Health, the Scottish Home and Health Department and the Welsh Office. They aim to provide up-to-date information about the prevalence of psychiatric problems among adults in Great Britain as well as their associated social disabilities and use of services.

Four separate surveys were carried out from April 1993 to August 1994.

i)   10,000 adults aged 16 to 64 years living in private households (fieldwork: April 1993– September 1993)

ii) a supplementary sample of 350 people aged 16 to 64 years with psychosis living in private households (fieldwork: October 1993 – December 1993)

iii) 1,200 people aged 16 to 64 years living in institutions specifically catering for people with mental illness (fieldwork: April 1994 – July 1994)

iv) 1,100 homeless people aged 16 to 64 years living in hostels for the homeless or other such institutions. This sample also included people sleeping rough (fieldwork July 1994 – August 1994)

The results of the surveys are being presented in a series of reports of which this is the first. This Report describes the main concepts and instruments common to all four surveys (Chapters 1 and 2) and presents specific information about the survey carried out in private households (Chapter 3) and the prevalence rates of disorders of people living in private households (Chapters 4, 5 and 6).

The main focus of the survey was neurotic psychopathology as measured by the Clinical Interview Schedule — Revised (CIS–R). This involved asking survey respondents about the presence of 14 symptoms in the past month, and their frequency, severity and duration in the past week. Attempts were also made to estimate the prevalence of psychosis, drug dependence and alcohol dependence. For psychosis, respondents were screened for reported psychotic features and possible sufferers were followed up with a clinical interview (SCAN). Alcohol and drug dependence were assessed from answers to a self-completion questionnaire.

The results of the survey are presented according to three levels of specificity: a broad measure based on a threshold score for neurotic psychopathology; one indicating a threshold score or higher for particular symptoms; and the prevalence of psychiatric disorders.

Neurotic psychopathology
(Chapter 4)

The survey revealed that overall about 1 in 7 adults aged 16 to 64 had some sort of neurotic heath problem (as measured by a score of 12 or more on the CIS–R) in the week prior to interview. The likelihood of such a score among the unemployed was twice that of working people. Other groups of adults with high scores were women, people living alone, those living in rented rather than owned accommodation, and urban rather than rural dwellers.

Neurotic symptoms (Chapter 5)

Of the fourteen symptoms covered by the CIS R, four stood out in both men and women.

These were fatigue (affecting 27% of respondents), sleep problems (25%), irritability (22%), and worry, not including worry about physical health (20%). Women were considerably more likely than men to have every symptom except worry about physical health, and married women had the lowest prevalence of these symptoms compared with other women. Among men, those who were separated, and to a lesser extent, widowed and divorced, had far higher rates of prevalence of most symptoms.

Unemployment was very strongly associated with the prevalence of almost all neurotic symptoms and of all the factors studied, it made the greatest difference in symptom prevalence, followed by economic inactivity (i.e. unemployed and not seeking work). The odds of having many of the symptoms were twice as high among unemployed people as those in full-time employment.

The type of family unit significantly affected the prevalence of almost all symptoms, especially in women. Lone parents and people living alone or without close relatives had the highest odds of having symptoms compared with people living in couples with no children. Having children increased the prevalence of many of the symptoms, notably irritability, but these effects were small among men.

Tenure and locality were also significant factors. Renters had the greatest prevalence of having most symptoms, often up to 50% higher than owner occupiers. There was a higher prevalence of many symptoms among those who rented from local authorities and housing associations compared with renters in the private sector. Living in an urban area was associated with a higher prevalence of most symptoms compared with living elsewhere; the odds of having many symptoms was 20–40% higher among people in urban areas.

Psychiatric disorders (Chapter 6)

The most prevalent neurotic disorder within the week prior to interview was mixed anxiety and depressive disorder (77 cases per thousand) followed by Generalised Anxiety Disorder (31 per thousand), depressive episode (21 per thousand), Obsessive Compulsive Disorder (12 per thousand), phobia (11 per thousand) and panic disorder (8 per thousand). The overall prevalence of neurotic disorder was 160 per thousand.

Three other psychiatric disorders were covered in the survey. Functional psychosis was found to have a prevalence of 4 per thousand in the past year. The overall rate of alcohol dependence was 47 per thousand, and of drug dependence, 22 per thousand (both in the past year).

Two factors were strongly related to psychiatric disorders. The first, employment status, was related to most disorders: compared with those working full time, the odds of having most disorders were more than doubled among unemployed and economically inactive people. The second factor, age, was particularly related to alcohol and drug dependence, with the odds of these disorders decreasing with age.

Family unit type and sex were also found to be related to psychiatric morbidity: being in a one-person family unit was particularly associated with increased odds of alcohol and drug dependency, and the odds of these disorders were also associated with being male. Compared to men, women had significantly increased odds of Generalised Anxiety Disorder and mixed anxiety and depressive disorder.

1 Background, aims and coverage of the survey

1.1 Background

Mental illness was identified as one of the five key areas for action in *The Health of the Nation*, a White Paper published by the Department of Health in July 1992.[1] The main target in this area was to improve significantly the health and social functioning of people with mental illness. To achieve this goal, it is necessary to have good baseline information about mental illness. In 1992, the Department of Health in conjunction with the Scottish Office and the Welsh Office, therefore commissioned OPCS to carry out a survey of psychiatric morbidity.

The OPCS survey is the first nationally representative survey of psychiatric morbidity to be carried out in Great Britain. There are several other sources of information about mental illness but these data are collected for specific purposes and have limited national applicability.[2] The Health of the Nation, Key Area Handbook on mental illness states why the available statistics may underestimate the extent of mental illness in the population.[3]

'the failure to recognise some mental illness at community and primary health care level.

the failure to recognise psychiatric morbidity in general medical and surgical settings.

insufficient attention given to psychological distress associated with physical diseases, particularly those associated with long term disablement, for both the patient and their carers.

the substantial effect of mental illness on other morbidity and mortality statistics and the under-reporting of mental illness due to stigma.'

The advantages of carrying out a large national survey of psychiatric morbidity among a representative sample of the population are that a concerted effort could be put into identifying people with mental health problems including those who had not been in contact with health, social and voluntary care services, and all informants could be asked the same questions in a standardised way and their answers recorded in the same systematic manner.

1.2 Aims of the survey

There were five main aims of the survey.

To estimate the prevalence of psychiatric morbidity
One of the main reasons for carrying out the survey was to estimate the prevalence of psychiatric morbidity according to diagnostic category and symptomatology among adults aged 16 to 64 years in Great Britain. Prevalence rates of symptoms as well as diagnoses have been calculated because of the relationship between the presence of symptoms, social disabilities and the need for services.

To identify social disabilities associated with mental illness
The survey aimed to identify the nature and extent of social disabilities associated with mental illness. Social disabilities refer to the limitations in function or restrictions in activities of people within particular environments: their homes, their workplace and their social relationships.

Service use
The varying use of services and the receipt of care are examined in relation to diagnosis, symptoms and their associated social disabilities.

1

To investigate recent stressful life events associated with mental illness

The focus was on how major stressful life events in the previous six months were related to how people were feeling at the time of the interview.

Lifestyles indicators

Another principal aim was to investigate the comorbidity between mental illness and smoking, drinking and drug use. As well as looking at the relationship between mental illness and tobacco, alcohol, and drug consumption, particular emphasis is put on the association between alcohol and drug dependency, and alcohol and drug-related problems, and the experience of mental illness.

1.3 Coverage of the survey

Region

The surveyed population comprised adults living in England, Wales and Scotland (excluding the Highlands and Islands).

Age

The survey focused on the prevalence of psychiatric morbidity among adults aged 16 to 64. Children, defined as those under the age of 16, were excluded from the survey as were adults aged 65 or above. This is because surveys of children's psychopathology and of psychiatric morbidity among elderly people would require specialised sampling, interviewing and assessment procedures.

Private households and institutions

The programme of psychiatric morbidity surveys included people living in institutions which specifically cater for people with mental illnesses as well as those living in private households[4, 5]. Adults aged 16 to 64 living in institutions represent a very small proportion of the total population but are likely to be extensive

consumers of health, social and voluntary care services. Although there is information about these residents, the survey offered an opportunity to classify them on the same instruments as those used for the private household survey.

1.4 Organisation of the survey (including timetable)

Private household surveys

The Postcode Address File (PAF) was chosen as the sampling frame for the first survey because it gives a good representation of private households in Great Britain. However, because very few people living in private households are likely to be suffering from a psychotic illness, a supplementary survey of people who were known to have a psychotic illness was required in order to achieve sufficient interviews to permit analysis of social disabilities and use of services among this group.

Institutional surveys

The surveys of residents in institutions were carried out as separate exercises from the private household surveys although the aim was to obtain as much comparable information as possible. The institutional surveys required a separate sampling design, a strategy to negotiate access to the establishment and the residents, and the use of modified questionnaires.[6]

Homeless people were targeted because previous research has shown that this group has a particularly high prevalence of major psychiatric morbidity - estimates vary from 30% to 50%.[7] Institutions which cater for homeless people include private short leased accommodation, hostels for the homeless, day centres and night shelters. Some people sleeping rough were identified via their contact with day centres.[8]

1.5 Coverage of the current report

The main purpose of this Report is to present prevalence rates of psychiatric morbidity among adults aged 16 to 64 living in private households in Great Britain. In order to interpret these results, it is important to have an understanding of the conceptual approach and methods adopted for this study, and these are described in Chapters 2 and 3.

The main results are presented in Chapters 4 to 6. Chapters 4 and 5 focus on neurosis and neurotic symptoms whilst the following chapter covers the prevalence of neurotic disorders, functional psychoses, and alcohol and drug dependence.

1.6 Plans for later reports

Because of the ambitious nature of the programme of research and the sequential timetables for the four surveys, it is intended to produce a series of reports on different topics or populations, of which this is the first. This means that the early reports can be produced before all the survey analysis is complete and those interested in specific topics can refer to the relevant report.

The full set of results from the OPCS survey of psychiatric morbidity among adults aged 16 to 64 will be presented in a series of eight reports and four bulletins published in 1995. The content of these reports and bulletins are summarised below in the order of the planned publication schedule. Relevant questionnaires, and further methodological details will be included as appendices to the main reports.

Private household survey

Bulletin No. 1
Prevalence of psychiatric morbidity.

Report 1
Prevalence of psychiatric morbidity by socio-

demographic correlates; comorbidity among psychiatric disorders.

Report 2
Characteristics of people with mental disorders, medication and other forms of treatment, service use, and patient satisfaction with treatment and services.

Report 3
Difficulties associated with mental disorders in respect of activities of daily living, employment, social functioning, finances. Recent stressful life events and lifestyle behaviours (use of tobacco, alcohol and drugs and their consequences).

Institutions survey

Bulletin No. 2
Prevalence of psychiatric morbidity in institutions.

Report 4
Prevalence of psychiatric morbidity by type of institution; comorbidity among psychiatric disorders.

Report 5
Characteristics of people with mental disorders living in institutions, medication, other forms of treatment, and service use within and outside the institution; patient satisfaction with treatment and services.

Report 6
Difficulties associated with mental disorders in respect of activities of daily living, employment, social functioning, finances. Recent stressful life events and lifestyle behaviours (use of tobacco, alcohol and drugs and their consequences).

Survey of homeless people

Bulletin No. 3
Prevalence of psychiatric morbidity among homeless people.

Report 7

Prevalence of psychiatric morbidity by type of 'accommodation'; medication, other forms of treatment, and service use; difficulties associated with mental disorders in respect of housing, activities of daily living, employment, social functioning, finances. Recent stressful life events and lifestyle behaviours (use of tobacco, alcohol and drugs and their consequences).

People suffering from a psychotic illness

Bulletin No. 4

Summary of the characteristics of people with psychosis.

Report 8

Profiles of people with psychosis in terms of differential use of treatment and services.

Access to the data

Anonymised data from all four surveys will be lodged with the ESRC Data Archive, University of Essex, within three months of the publication of the main reports.[9]

Notes and references

1. *The Health of the Nation: A Strategy for Health in England*, DH, HMSO, 1992.

2. *Public Health Information Strategy: Improving Information on Mental health*, DH, May 1993, Appendix A1, page 29.

3. *The Health of the Nation: Key Area Handbook on Mental Illness*, DH, 1993, Section 1.5, page 12.

4. The distinction is made between institutions and private households in preference to institutions and community.

5. Inmates of prisons, and residents of military, educational and religious establishments have been excluded from the coverage of the survey.

6. Details of the sampling and interviewing procedures for the institutional surveys will be found in Report 4 of the OPCS series of reports on psychiatric morbidity.

7. Scott, J. (1993) Review article: Homelessness and mental illness *British Journal of Psychiatry*, **162**: 314-25.

8. Further details of the survey of psychiatric morbidity among homeless people are found in Report 7.

9. Independent researchers who wish to carry out their own analyses should apply to the Archive for access. For further information about archived data please contact:

MS Kathy Sayer
ESRC Data Archive
University of Essex
Wivenhoe Park
Colchester
Essex CO4 3SQ

Tel: (UK) 01206 872323
Fax: (UK)01206 872003
Email: archive@: Essex. AC. UK.

2 Measurement and classification of psychiatric disorders

2.1 Choice of measurement instruments

Two different research strategies were used to obtain prevalence estimates of psychiatric morbidity. One approach was used for the relatively numerous, minor psychiatric disorders (neurotic psychopathology), the other was required for the less frequently occurring major psychiatric disorders (psychotic psychopathology).

2.1.1 Neurotic psychopathology

To obtain the prevalence of both symptoms and diagnoses of neurotic psychopathology, the revised version of the Clinical Interview Schedule (CIS-R) was chosen.[1] Lewis gives the rationale for its use:

'Many of the standardised interviews currently used in psychiatry require the interviewer to use expert psychiatric judgements in deciding upon the presence or absence of psychopathology. However, when case definitions are standardised it is customary for clinical judgements to be replaced with rules. The Clinical Interview Schedule was therefore revised, in order to increase standardisation, and to make it suitable for lay interviewers in assessing minor psychiatric disorder in community, general hospital, occupational and primary care research'

The practical advantages of the CIS-R are:

- it can be administered by non-clinically trained interviewers

- training in the use of the schedule is straightforward for experienced OPCS interviewers

- length of interview is relatively short (on average, 30 minutes) compared with other methods of assessment.

The CIS-R is made up of fourteen sections, each section covering a particular area of neurotic symptoms.

The fourteen sections of the CIS–R

Fatigue
Sleep problems
Irritability
Worry (excluding worry about physical health)
Depression
Depressive ideas
Anxiety
Obsessions
Concentration and forgetfulness
Somatic symptoms
Compulsions
Phobias
Worry about physical health
Panic

Each section within the interview schedule starts with a variable number of mandatory questions which can be regarded as sift or filter questions. They establish the existence of a particular neurotic symptom in the past month. A positive response to these questions leads the interviewer on to further enquiry giving a more detailed assessment of the symptom in the past week: frequency, duration, severity and time since onset. It is the answers to these questions which determine the informant's score on each section. More frequent and more severe symptoms result in higher scores.

The minimum score on each section is 0, where the symptom was either not present in the past week or was present only in mild degree. The maximum score on each section is 4 (except for the section on Depressive ideas which has a maximum score of 5).

- Summed scores from all 14 sections range between 0 and 57.

- The overall threshold score for significant psychiatric morbidity is 12.

- Symptoms are regarded as severe if they have a score of 2 or more.

For each symptom the elements which contribute to a score are shown in Appendix B, Part 1. As an illustration, the elements which contribute to a score on the section on Anxiety are shown below.

Calculation of symptom score for Anxiety from the CIS-R

	Score
Felt **generally** anxious/nervous/tense for **4 days or more** in the past seven days	1
In past seven days anxiety/nervousness/ tension has been **very unpleasant**	1
In the past seven days have felt **any of the following symptoms** when anxious/nervous/tense (racing heart, sweating or shaking hands, feeling dizzy, difficulty getting one's breath, dry mouth, butterflies in stomach, nausea or wanting to vomit)	1
Felt anxious/nervous/tense for **more than three hours** in total on any one of the past seven days	1

Any combination of the elements produce the section score.

Diagnoses are obtained by looking at the answers to various sections, including questions which do not necessarily score points, and applying algorithms based on ICD-10 diagnostic criteria.[2] The algorithms for all disorders are shown in Appendix B, Part 2 and the example that follows is for Generalised Anxiety Disorder (GAD).

Algorithm for GAD

Conditions which must apply are:

- Duration greater than six months
- Free-floating anxiety
- Autonomic overactivity
- Overall score on Anxiety section was 2 or more

2.1.2 Psychotic psychopathology

Making assessments of psychotic rather than neurotic disorders is more problematic for lay interviewers. A structured questionnaire is too restrictive and a semi-structured questionnaire requires the use of clinical judgements. Therefore OPCS interviewers were only asked to carry out an initial, general investigation: was there any possibility of the subject suffering from a psychotic illness? Psychiatrists were used to carry out a follow-up clinical interview.

Because people who suffer from a psychotic illness are so rare in the private household population, the questions for the initial investigation were pitched at such a level to reduce as far as possible the number of false negatives at some cost of increasing the false positive rate.

Screening for psychosis included asking about presently occurring symptoms, but also asking informants directly what was the matter with them; whether they were taking anti-psychotic drugs or having anti-psychotic injections, and whether they had contact with any health care professional for a mental, nervous or emotional problem which had been labelled as a psychotic illness. The sift for presently occurring symptoms, Psychosis Screening Questionnaire (PSQ), was developed specifically for this project.[3] The additional questions were added to minimise the false negative rate in the context of a disorder of low prevalence.

Clinicians who followed up potential cases were trained to carry out their interviews using SCAN (Schedules for Clinical Assessment in Neuropsychiatry) which is programmed on to a lap-top computer.[45] SCAN is a set of instruments aimed at assessing, measuring and classifying the psychopathology and behaviour associated with the major psychiatric disorders of adult life. Of its four main components, the PSE10, was the one deemed most applicable for the purposes of this survey.[6] The PSE10 itself has two parts. Part One covers, inter alia, anxiety, depressive and bipolar disorders. Part Two includes the psychotic disorders of interest to the survey (schizophrenia, schizotypal and other delusional disorders).

2.1.3 Alcohol and drug dependence

A measure of alcohol dependence was created from adding up positive responses to 12 questions which focus on the three components of dependence: loss of control, symptomatic behaviour and binge drinking. A score of three or more was defined as indicating alcohol dependence.

Five questions in the survey measured drug dependence: frequency of drug use, stated dependence, inability to cut down, need for larger amounts, and withdrawal symptoms. A positive response to any statement was used to indicate drug dependence.

A list of the specific questions which were used to assess alcohol and drug dependence are found in Appendix B, Part 3.

2.2 Classification of disorders

Instruments used for clinical assessments of psychiatric disorders often allow for several possible diagnoses to be made. The hierarchy adopted for this survey was that functional psychoses (schizophrenia and manic-depression) took precedence over the existence of other symptoms which would lead to a diagnosis of a neurotic disorder. In ICD-10 terms, F20–F39 took precedence over F40–F48. Alcohol and drug dependence were considered separately.

Within the six neurotic categories the rules in the table below were applied to obtain the dominant disorder:

Figure 2.1 shows how the overall ninefold classification of disorders was constructed.

Disorder 1	Disorder 2	Priority
Depressive episode (any severity)	Phobia	Depressive episode (any severity)
Depressive episode (mild)	OCD	OCD
Depressive episode (moderate)	OCD	Depressive episode (moderate)
Depressive episode (severe)	OCD	Depressive episode (severe)
Depressive episode (mild)	Panic disorder	Panic disorder
Depressive episode (moderate)	Panic disorder	Depressive episode (moderate)
Depressive episode (any severity)	GAD	Depressive episode (any severity)
Phobia (any)	OCD	OCD
Agoraphobia	GAD	Agoraphobia
Social phobia	GAD	Social phobia
Specific phobia	GAD	GAD
Panic disorder	OCD	Panic disorder
OCD	GAD	OCD
Panic disorder	GAD	Panic disorder

GAD = Generalised Anxiety Disorder; OCD = Obsessive– Compulsive Disorder

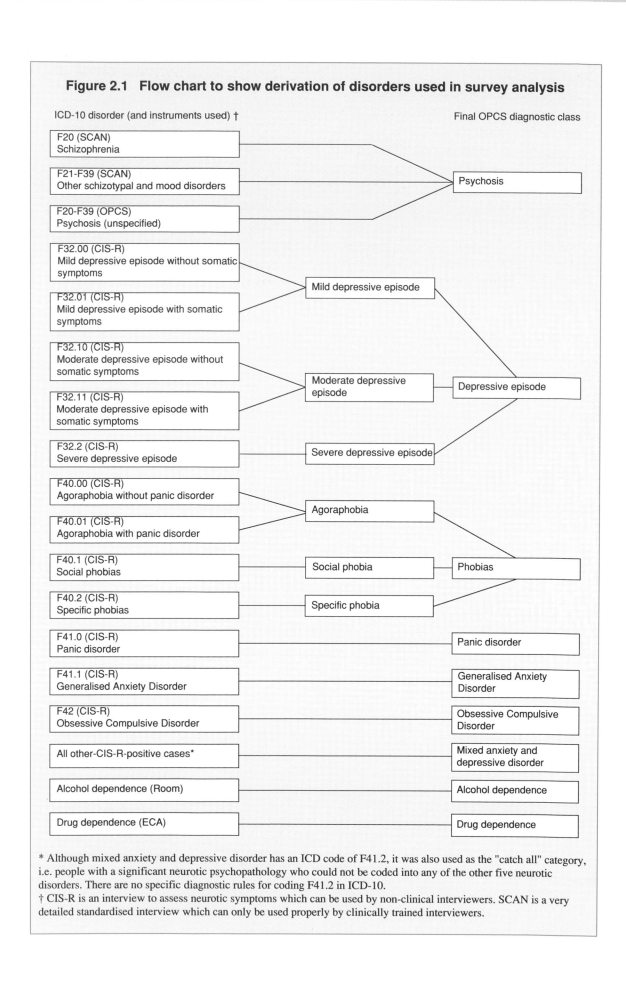

Figure 2.1 Flow chart to show derivation of disorders used in survey analysis

ICD-10 disorder (and instruments used) †

Final OPCS diagnostic class

F20 (SCAN)
Schizophrenia

F21-F39 (SCAN)
Other schizotypal and mood disorders

F20-F39 (OPCS)
Psychosis (unspecified)

Psychosis

F32.00 (CIS-R)
Mild depressive episode without somatic symptoms

F32.01 (CIS-R)
Mild depressive episode with somatic symptoms

Mild depressive episode

F32.10 (CIS-R)
Moderate depressive episode without somatic symptoms

F32.11 (CIS-R)
Moderate depressive episode with somatic symptoms

Moderate depressive episode

Depressive episode

F32.2 (CIS-R)
Severe depressive episode

Severe depressive episode

F40.00 (CIS-R)
Agoraphobia without panic disorder

F40.01 (CIS-R)
Agoraphobia with panic disorder

Agoraphobia

F40.1 (CIS-R)
Social phobias

Social phobia

Phobias

F40.2 (CIS-R)
Specific phobias

Specific phobia

F41.0 (CIS-R)
Panic disorder

Panic disorder

F41.1 (CIS-R)
Generalised Anxiety Disorder

Generalised Anxiety Disorder

F42 (CIS-R)
Obsessive Compulsive Disorder

Obsessive Compulsive Disorder

All other-CIS-R-positive cases*

Mixed anxiety and depressive disorder

Alcohol dependence (Room)

Alcohol dependence

Drug dependence (ECA)

Drug dependence

* Although mixed anxiety and depressive disorder has an ICD code of F41.2, it was also used as the "catch all" category, i.e. people with a significant neurotic psychopathology who could not be coded into any of the other five neurotic disorders. There are no specific diagnostic rules for coding F41.2 in ICD-10.

† CIS-R is an interview to assess neurotic symptoms which can be used by non-clinical interviewers. SCAN is a very detailed standardised interview which can only be used properly by clinically trained interviewers.

Notes and references

1. Lewis, G. and Pelosi, A.J., *Manual of the Revised Clinical Interview Schedule, (CIS-R),* June 1990, Institute of Psychiatry. See also Lewis, G., Pelosi, A.J., Araya, R.C. and Dunn, G., (1992) Measuring Psychiatric disorder in the community: a standardized assessment for use by lay interviewers, *Psychological Medicine*, **22**, 465-486.

2. *The ICD-10 Classification of Mental and Behavioural Disorders: Diagnostic Criteria for Research*: 1993, WHO, Geneva.

3. Bebbington, P.E., and Nayani, T (1994) The Psychosis Screening Questionnaire, *International Journal of Methods in Psychiatric Research*. (in press)

4. *Schedules for Clinical Assessment in Neuropsychiatry*, 1992, WHO, Division of Mental Health, Geneva.

5. Wing, J.K., Babor, T., Brugha, T., Burke, J., Cooper, J.E., Giel, R., Jablensky, A., Regier, D., and Sartorius, N. (1990) SCAN: Schedules for Clinical assessment in Neuropsychiatry *Archives of General Psychiatry*, **47,** 586-593.

6. Wing, J.K., Nixon, J., Mann, S.A., and Leff, J.P. (1977) Reliability of the PSE used in a population survey. *Psychological Medicine*, **7**: 505-516.

3 Sampling and interviewing procedures

3.1 Introduction

This and all subsequent chapters of this Report focus on the survey of psychiatric morbidity among adults aged 16 to 64 years living in private households.

3.2 Sampling procedures

The small users Postcode Address File (PAF) was chosen as the sampling frame because of its good coverage of private households in Great Britain. In the PAF, postal sectors were stratified by socio-economic group within Regional Health Authority. A postal sector has on average 2,550 delivery points.

Initially, 200 postal sectors were selected (the primary sampling units) with probability proportional to size (number of delivery points). Within each of the 200 postal sectors, 90 delivery points were selected, yielding a sample of 18,000 delivery points. This sample design was developed to produce precise, nationally representative prevalence rates, and to avoid 'contamination effects' due to heavy clustering.[1]

Interviewers visited these 18,000 addresses all over England, Scotland and Wales to identify private households with at least one person aged 16 to 64. The Kish grid method was used to select systematically one person in each household.[2]

3.3 Organisation of the interview

Every sampled adult was asked Schedule A which covered:[3]

- Socio-demographic characteristics
- General health questions
- Clinical Interview Schedule — Revised (CIS-R)
- The Psychosis Screening Questionnaire (PSQ) and associated questions which indicate the possibility of psychotic disorders

Individuals who were at or above the threshold on the CIS-R (a score of 12 or more) and those who gave indications of having a psychotic illness were asked Schedule B which was made up of ten sections:

- Long standing illness
- Medication and treatment
- Health, Social and Voluntary care services
- Activities of daily living and informal care
- Recent stressful life events factors
- Social activities, social networks and social support
- Education and employment
- Finances
- Smoking
- Alcohol consumption

Those below the threshold were asked Schedule C, an abridged version of Schedule B, in order to get comparable information on topics where there were no published national data. Because these informants were assumed to have no mental health problems, the questionnaire was shortened by omitting the sections on long standing illness, medication and treatment, and use of services.

All subjects were given a self completion questionnaire covering alcohol dependency and problems, drug-taking, and dependency and problems as a result of the use of drugs.

Subjects who were found by the OPCS

interviewer potentially to be suffering from a psychotic illness were followed up within a few weeks by a psychiatrist who conducted a clinical interview.

The path through the different interview schedules is shown in Figure 3.1.

3.4 Results of the sampling procedures

Twelve per cent of addresses were ineligible because they contained no private households. Of the private household addresses 23% contained no-one within the eligible age range

Table 3.1 Households eligible for interivew

	No.	%
Sample of addresses	**18,000**	**100**
Vacant premises	927	5
Institution/business premises	573	3
Demolished	499	3
Second home/holiday flat	236	1
Private household addresses	**15,765**	**88**
Private household addresses	**15,765**	
Extra households found	669	
Total number of households	16,434	100
Household with no one aged 16-64	3,704	23
Households eligible for interview	**12,730**	**77**

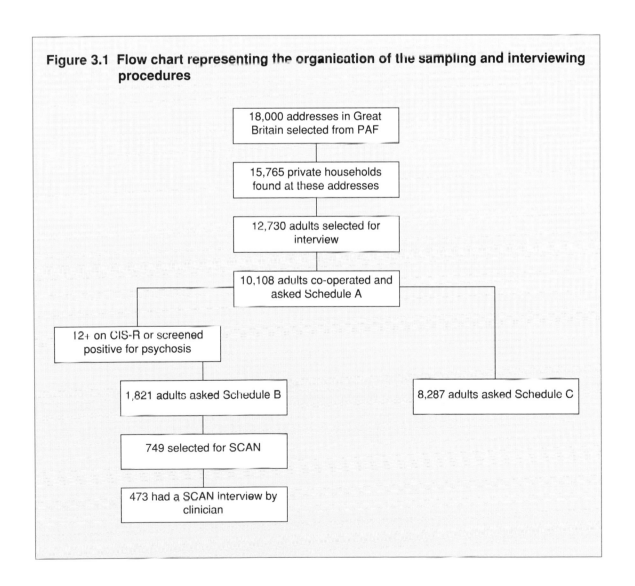

Figure 3.1 Flow chart representing the organisation of the sampling and interviewing procedures

18,000 addresses in Great Britain selected from PAF

15,765 private households found at these addresses

12,730 adults selected for interview

10,108 adults co-operated and asked Schedule A

12+ on CIS-R or screened positive for psychosis

1,821 adults asked Schedule B

8,287 adults asked Schedule C

749 selected for SCAN

473 had a SCAN interview by clinician

(*Table 3.1*). Four out of five people selected for interview agreed to be interviewed (*Table 3.2*).

Table 3.2 Response of adults at interview stage

	No.	%
Set sample of households	**12,730**	**100**
Refusals	1,641	13
Non contacts	981	8
Co-operating adults	10,108	80

3.5 Interviewing procedures

Pre-pilot and pilot surveys

Before carrying out the main stage survey of psychiatric morbidity in private households, one pre-pilot and three pilot surveys were carried out. The aim of these exercises was not only to validate our instruments but also to test the reaction to the survey among the general population, and to refine the question order and content. The largest pilot exercise involved 1,000 people.

Organisation and training of interviewers

Two hundred interviewers were personally briefed for the private household survey. These interviewers were part of the OPCS general field force, and had already been trained in the same way to a high standard to work on government sponsored surveys. Those with least experience had 'trainers' allocated to them to ensure that the proper standards were reached.

Interviewers were each given 90 addresses divided into two quotas of 45 addresses. Interviewers were asked to complete each quota within 6 weeks with a break of a month between quotas.

Maximising response

In order to maximise cooperation, letters were sent to sampled addresses explaining the purpose of the survey and that an interviewer would call.

In addition, interviewers made several calls at an address, if necessary, to make contact.

Introducing the survey

Interviewers were briefed on how to introduce the survey on the doorstep. They were told to avoid using terms such as 'psychiatric morbidity' or 'mental illness'. The results from our pilot surveys indicated that most people could relate to the expressions 'health and well-being' and 'coping with the stresses and strains of everyday life'. The four main points covered in the introduction were:

(a) who the survey was for
(b) what the survey was about
(c) how the results would be used
(d) how their address was sampled

Proxy information

In some circumstances proxy information was collected, rather than lose information about the selected informant. This was especially relevant when the subject could not answer questions due to a mental health problem, but also applied to informants who were too physically ill, had a speech or hearing problem, or had language problems.

The nature of the Clinical Interview Schedule does not readily permit the use of an interpreter for informants who have problems understanding English. This is because many of the concepts do not have equivalent terms in other languages. In such circumstances proxy interviews were carried out.

Notes and references

1. Contamination in this respect means that people who have been interviewed talk to those yet to be interviewed and influence their answers.

2. A full explanation of the Kish grid for sampling is given in Appendix A.

3. See Appendix C.

4 Distribution of CIS-R scores

4.1 Introduction

In this chapter the results of using the Clinical Interview Schedule — Revised to question approximately 10,000 adults are presented. The focus is on the relationship between the overall score on the CIS-R and various characteristics of informants.

Figure 4.1 shows the distribution of total scores on the CIS-R for the surveyed sample and illustrates that 14% of the sample were on or above the threshold score of 12. Among those below the threshold most had a score of less than 6: two thirds of the total sample.

Throughout the chapter, tables show data separately for women and men and then for all adults. Women were more likely than men to have a CIS-R score which was on or above the threshold score of 12, i.e. to have significant, neurotic psychopathology *(Figure 4.2)*.

The final section of the chapter, 4.7, presents odds ratios of socio-demographic correlates of the CIS-R score; these show which of the personal, family and household characteristics presented in the preceding sections were most strongly associated with CIS-R scores.

4.2 Distribution of the CIS-R score by personal characteristics

Age

The proportions of adults with a score of 12 or more varied little between the ages of 20 and 54, about 12% for men and 20% for women. Those with the smallest proportions at or above the threshold were men aged 16 to 19 (6%) and women aged 60 to 64 (10%) *(Table 4.1)*

Ethnicity

The distribution of CIS-R scores by ethnicity is difficult to interpret because only 4% of the sample classified themselves as belonging to the West Indian, African, Asian or Oriental ethnic groups and 1% would not classify themselves into any ethnic group. Nevertheless,

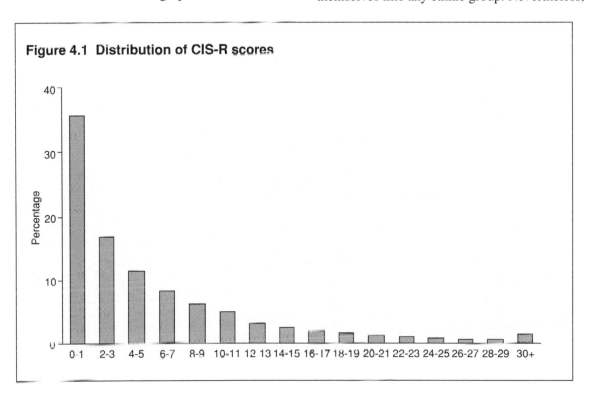

Figure 4.1 Distribution of CIS-R scores

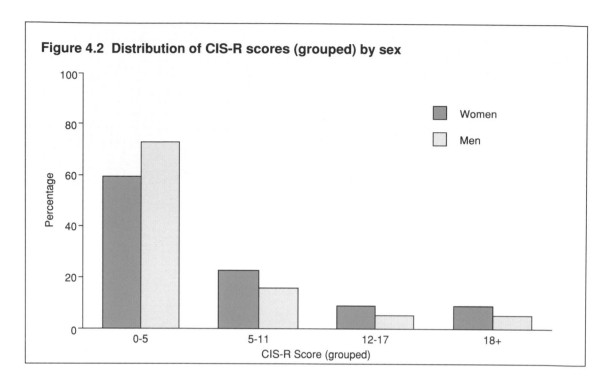

Figure 4.2 Distribution of CIS-R scores (grouped) by sex

the data do indicate a slightly smaller proportion of Whites than of other ethnic groups with scores of 12 or more. Differences in the distributions of CIS-R scores between men and womem occurred for all ethnic groups. (*Table 4.2*)

Marital status

Marital status had a marked association with neurotic psychopathology for both men and women. The groups with the highest CIS-R scores were divorced and separated women, and men who were separated from their wives; almost thirty per cent of these three groups had a score of 12 or more. They were three times more likely than single, married and cohabiting men to exhibit significant neurotic symptoms. (*Table 4.3*)

Education

The overall score on the CIS-R was unrelated to the age at which individuals left full-time education or to their highest educational qualifications. (*Tables 4.4 and 4.5*)

Employment

Employment status was highly correlated with

expressed neurotic symptoms with unemployed men and women having high CIS-R scores. About one in four of all unemployed adults and one in five of the economically inactive had an overall CIS-R score of 12 or more. Men who were not working were twice as likely as working men to exhibit significant neurotic psychopathology. However, the group with the highest CIS-R scores of all, were women who were not working and were seeking work: 37% had a CIS-R score of 12 or more. (*Table 4.6*)

Social class

Among men, those in Social Class I (Professionals) were less prone to have neurotic symptoms than all others. Among women, those in Social Class II (Employers and managers) joined those in Social Class I as having the lowest proportions with a score on or above the threshold. (*Table 4.7*)

4.3 Distribution of the CIS-R score by family characteristics

Family unit type

Relationships were found between the type of family unit people lived in, and having neurotic symptoms. Just over a quarter of lone parents (27%) had a score of 12 or more, compared with 14% of couples with children. This relationship was evident for both men and women. About one in five adults living alone experienced severe neurotic symptoms in the week prior to interview. Adults living with parents were least likely to have CIS-R scores of 12 or more (9%). *(Table 4.8)*

4.4 Distribution of the CIS-R score by household characteristics

Tenure and type of accommodation

People living in accommodation rented from local authorities or housing associations were twice as likely to have experienced severe neurotic symptoms in the past week as those living in owned or mortgaged properties (22% compared with 11%). There was little difference between outright owners and mortgagees. Seventeen per cent of those living in private rented accommodation had CIS-R scores of 12 or more, a lower proportion than among those renting from local authorities, but a higher proportion than was found among the group living in owned or mortgaged properties. *(Table 4.9)*

About one in five occupants of terraced properties, maisonettes or flats had experienced severe neurotic symptoms in the past week compared with one in eight people living in detached or semi-detached properties. A higher proportion of women with neurotic psychopathology was evident in all situations. *(Table 4.10)*

Ownership of a car or van

Whether a household has a car or van, and the number of such vehicles available, is an indicator of socio-economic status and this gave the clearest picture of the relationship between socio-economic status and neurotic psychopathology. Men and women living in households without the use of a car or van were twice as likely to score 12 or more on the CIS-R as those

in households with three or more cars (22% compared with 10%). *(Table 4.11)*

4.5 Distribution of the CIS-R score by personal and household characteristics combined

By looking at several personal and household characteristics at the same time, it is possible to produce a hierarchy from the most to the least vulnerable groups. The comparison by sex is retained as this has been shown in all previous tables to be a key variable in differentiating high from low weekly prevalence rates of neurotic symptoms.

The four factors considered together are type of accommodation, tenure, employment status and marital status. Table 4.12 shows that all these factors had an additive effect in determining high CIS-R scores. The combination of single, widowed, separated or divorced women, not working and living in a rented, terraced house, flat or maisonette produced the highest level of neurotic psychopathology, 34%. The lowest proportions (5% and 7%) were found among single and married men who were working, and living in a house bought outright or with a mortgage. *(Table 4.12)*

4.6 Distribution of the CIS-R score by region and locality

Country and Region

The proportions of adults with a score of 12 or more were very similar in England, Scotland and Wales (16-17%).

When the survey took place, there were 14 Regional Health Authorities (RHAs) in existence. Scotland and Wales were regarded as distinct regions, making 16 regions in all. There were small differences in the distributions of CIS-R scores between most regions. There were, however, one or two regions which had marked differences from the other regions.

15

Among men living in East Anglia RHA, just 6% had a score of 12 or more on the CIS-R, the smallest proportion among all RHAs. The two regions which stood out for women were North East Thames and Mersey; both had 26% of women with a CIS-R score of 12 or more. *(Table 4.13)*

Locality

Living in an urban rather than a rural locality was associated with a higher proportion of both men and women with CIS-R scores on or above the threshold score of 12. The proportion of men in urban areas having such scores was double that of men in rural localities. Women living in urban areas were also more likely to have a CIS-R score on or above the threshold than those living in a semi-rural locality. *(Table 4.14)*

4.7 Odds ratios of socio-demographic correlates of the overall CIS-R score

Logistic regression was undertaken to provide a measure of the effect of various socio-demographic variables on CIS-R scores and odds ratios were produced. Appendix D explains the way in which this analysis was carried out.

Table 4.15 shows that after controlling for the nine other personal, family and household characteristics, being unemployed was the most significant correlate of a high CIS-R score, with an odds ratio of 2.26 compared with those working full time. Lone parents were 56% more likely than married couples to have a score of 12 or more, the same odds ratios for women compared with men . *(Table 4.15)*

Table 4.1   CIS-R score (grouped) by age and sex (SE in brackets)

CIS-R score	Age										All
	16-19	20-24	25-29	30-34	35-39	40-44	45-49	50-54	55-59	60-64	
	%	%	%	%	%	%	%	%	%	%	%
Women											
0-5	59 (3)	54 (3)	57 (2)	56 (2)	60 (2)	56 (2)	62 (2)	60 (2)	65 (2)	69 (2)	59 (1)
6-11	25 (3)	26 (2)	25 (2)	23 (2)	21 (2)	24 (2)	20 (2)	19 (2)	21 (2)	20 (2)	23 (1)
Under 12	**84 (2)**	**80 (2)**	**82 (2)**	**79 (2)**	**81 (2)**	**80 (2)**	**82 (2)**	**79 (2)**	**86 (2)**	**89 (1)**	**82 (1)**
12-17	6 (2)	11 (1)	9 (1)	11 (1)	8 (1)	9 (1)	10 (1)	10 (1)	7 (1)	6 (1)	9 (0)
18+	10 (2)	10 (1)	8 (1)	10 (1)	11 (1)	10 (1)	9 (1)	12 (2)	6 (1)	4 (1)	9 (1)
12 or above	**16 (2)**	**21 (2)**	**17 (2)**	**21 (2)**	**19 (2)**	**19 (2)**	**19 (2)**	**22 (2)**	**13 (2)**	**10 (1)**	**18 (1)**
Base	*365*	*555*	*648*	*587*	*531*	*529*	*520*	*413*	*396*	*390*	*4933*
Men											
0-5	77 (3)	73 (2)	73 (2)	70 (2)	72 (2)	68 (2)	74 (2)	77 (2)	74 (2)	75 (2)	73 (1)
6-11	18 (3)	17 (2)	15 (2)	18 (2)	15 (1)	20 (2)	15 (2)	12 (2)	14 (2)	14 (2)	16 (1)
Under 12	**94 (2)**	**90 (1)**	**88 (1)**	**88 (1)**	**87 (1)**	**88 (2)**	**89 (2)**	**89 (2)**	**88 (2)**	**89 (2)**	**89 (1)**
12-17	1 (1)	7 (1)	6 (1)	8 (1)	5 (1)	6 (1)	4 (1)	5 (1)	6 (1)	6 (1)	6 (0)
18+	4 (1)	4 (1)	6 (1)	4 (1)	7 (1)	6 (1)	7 (1)	5 (1)	7 (1)	5 (1)	6 (0)
12 or above	**6 (2)**	**11 (1)**	**12 (1)**	**12 (1)**	**12 (1)**	**12 (2)**	**11 (2)**	**10 (2)**	**13 (2)**	**11 (2)**	**12 (0)**
Base	*382*	*569*	*651*	*575*	*505*	*500*	*501*	*415*	*387*	*374*	*4859*
All adults											
0-5	68 (2)	63 (2)	65 (2)	63 (2)	66 (2)	62 (2)	68 (1)	68(2)	69 (2)	72 (2)	66 (1)
6-11	21 (2)	22 (2)	20 (1)	20 (1)	18 (1)	22 (1)	18 (1)	16 (1)	17 (1)	17 (1)	19 (1)
Under 12	**89 (2)**	**85 (1)**	**85 (1)**	**83 (1)**	**84 (1)**	**84 (1)**	**86 (1)**	**84 (1)**	**86 (1)**	**89 (1)**	**85 (0)**
12-17	4 (1)	9 (1)	8 (1)	9 (1)	7 (1)	8 (1)	7 (1)	8 (1)	7 (1)	6 (1)	7 (0)
18+	7 (1)	6 (1)	7 (1)	7 (1)	9 (1)	8 (1)	8 (1)	8 (1)	6 (1)	5 (1)	7 (0)
12 or above	**11 (2)**	**15 (1)**	**15 (1)**	**16 (1)**	**16 (1)**	**16 (1)**	**15 (1)**	**16 (1)**	**13 (1)**	**11 (1)**	**14 (0)**
Base	*747*	*1124*	*1298*	*1161*	*1036*	*1029*	*1021*	*828*	*782*	*765*	*9792*

Table 4.2   CIS-R score (grouped) by ethnicity and sex (SE in brackets)

CIS-R score	Ethnicity *			All
	White	West Indian or African	Asian or Oriental	
	%	%	%	%
Women				
0-5	59 (1)	56 (5)	58 (7)	59 (1)
6-11	23 (1)	22 (4)	18 (4)	23 (1)
Under 12	**82 (1)**	**78 (4)**	**76 (5)**	**81 (1)**
12-17	9 (1)	14 (3)	13 (4)	9 (0)
18+	9 (1)	8 (3)	11 (3)	9 (1)
12 or above	**18 (1)**	**22 (4)**	**24 (5)**	**18 (1)**
Base	*4633*	*78*	*141*	*4933*
Men				
0-5	73 (1)	64 (7)	81 (4)	73 (1)
6-11	16 (1)	20 (5)	8 (3)	16 (1)
Under 12	**89 (1)**	**84 (4)**	**89 (3)**	**89 (1)**
12-17	6 (0)	3 (1)	4 (2)	6 (0)
18+	5 (0)	13 (4)	8 (3)	6 (0)
12 or above	**11 (1)**	**16 (4)**	**12 (3)**	**12 (1)**
Base	*4546*	*70*	*158*	*4859*
All adults				
0-5	66 (1)	60 (5)	70 (4)	66 (1)
6-11	20 (1)	21 (3)	13 (2)	19 (1)
Under 12	**86 (0)**	**81 (3)**	**83 (3)**	**85 (0)**
12-17	7 (0)	9 (2)	8 (2)	7 (0)
18+	7 (0)	10 (3)	9 (2)	7 (0)
12 or above	**14 (0)**	**19 (3)**	**17 (3)**	**14 (0)**
Base	*9179*	*148*	*299*	*9792*

* Respondents who could not be classified into the three ethnic groups or refused to answer are included in the "All" category.

Table 4.3   CIS-R score (grouped) by marital status and sex (SE in brackets)

CIS-R score	Marital status*						All
	Married	Cohabiting	Single	Widowed	Divorced	Separated	
	%	%	%	%	%	%	%
Women							
0-5	63 (1)	50 (3)	57 (2)	55 (3)	50 (3)	53 (4)	59 (1)
6-11	22 (1)	27 (3)	24 (2)	23 (3)	21 (2)	22 (3)	23 (1)
Under 12	**85 (1)**	**77 (2)**	**81 (1)**	**78 (3)**	**71 (2)**	**75 (3)**	**82 (1)**
12-17	8 (1)	12 (2)	8 (1)	10 (2)	13 (2)	10 (2)	9 (0)
18+	7 (1)	12 (2)	10 (1)	12 (2)	16 (2)	16 (3)	9 (1)
12 or above	**15 (1)**	**24 (2)**	**18 (1)**	**22 (3)**	**29 (2)**	**26 (3)**	**18 (1)**
Base	*2927*	*362*	*1014*	*171*	*314*	*127*	*4933*
Men							
0-5	74 (1)	70 (3)	73 (2)	66 (7)	67 (3)	55 (6)	73 (1)
6-11	15 (1)	20 (2)	16 (1)	14 (5)	16 (2)	16 (3)	16 (1)
Under 12	**89 (1)**	**90 (2)**	**89 (1)**	**80 (5)**	**83 (2)**	**71 (6)**	**89 (1)**
12-17	5 (0)	5 (1)	6 (1)	14 (5)	9 (2)	9 (3)	5 (0)
18+	6 (0)	6 (1)	4 (1)	6 (3)	8 (1)	20 (4)	6 (0)
12 or above	**11 (1)**	**11 (2)**	**10 (1)**	**20 (5)**	**17 (2)**	**29 (6)**	**11 (1)**
Base	*2868*	*327*	*1343*	*42*	*196*	*56*	*4859*
All adults							
0-5	68 (1)	59 (2)	66 (1)	57 (3)	56 (2)	53 (3)	66 (1)
6-11	18 (1)	24 (2)	20 (1)	22 (3)	19 (2)	20 (2)	19 (1)
Under 12	**86 (1)**	**83 (1)**	**86 (1)**	**79 (2)**	**75 (2)**	**73 (3)**	**85 (0)**
12-17	7 (0)	8 (1)	7 (1)	11 (2)	12 (1)	10 (2)	7 (0)
18+	6 (0)	9 (1)	7 (1)	10 (2)	13 (1)	17 (2)	7 (0)
12 or above	**13 (1)**	**17 (1)**	**14 (1)**	**21 (2)**	**25 (2)**	**27 (3)**	**14 (0)**
Base	*5795*	*688*	*2357*	*213*	*510*	*183*	*9792*

* Respondents with insufficient information to code marital status are included in the "All" category.

Table 4.4 CIS-R score (grouped) by age when finished full-time education and sex (SE in brackets)

CIS-R score	Age when finished full-time education*							All
	Not yet finished	14 or under	15	16	17	18	19 or over	
	%	%	%	%	%	%	%	%
Women								
0-5	56 (4)	60 (2)	57 (2)	60 (1)	61 (2)	59 (2)	60 (2)	59 (1)
6-11	25 (4)	20 (2)	22 (1)	22 (1)	23 (2)	27 (2)	24 (2)	23 (1)
Under 12	**81 (3)**	**80 (2)**	**79 (1)**	**82 (1)**	**84 (2)**	**86 (2)**	**84 (1)**	**82 (1)**
12-17	6 (2)	10 (2)	10 (1)	9 (1)	8 (1)	8 (1)	9 (1)	9 (0)
18+	13 (3)	10 (2)	12 (1)	8 (1)	8 (1)	6 (1)	7 (1)	9 (1)
12 or above	**19 (3)**	**20 (2)**	**22 (1)**	**17 (1)**	**16 (2)**	**14 (2)**	**16 (1)**	**18 (1)**
Base	*241*	*346*	*1135*	*1498*	*496*	*464*	*744*	*4933*
Men								
0-5	70 (4)	73 (2)	69 (2)	75 (1)	78 (2)	76 (3)	73 (2)	73 (1)
6-11	20 (3)	13 (2)	18 (1)	15 (1)	15 (2)	14 (2)	17 (2)	16 (1)
Under 12	**89 (2)**	**86 (2)**	**87 (1)**	**90 (1)**	**93 (1)**	**90 (2)**	**90 (1)**	**89 (1)**
12-17	2 (1)	6 (1)	5 (1)	6 (1)	4 (1)	7 (2)	6 (1)	5 (0)
18+	8 (2)	8 (1)	7 (1)	5 (0)	3 (1)	3 (1)	5 (1)	6 (0)
12 or above	**10 (2)**	**14 (2)**	**12 (1)**	**11 (1)**	**7 (1)**	**10 (2)**	**11 (1)**	**11 (1)**
Base	*271*	*354*	*1100*	*1559*	*380*	*339*	*846*	*4859*
All adults								
0-5	63 (3)	66 (2)	63 (1)	68 (1)	69 (2)	66 (2)	67 (2)	66 (1)
6-11	22 (3)	17 (1)	20 (1)	18 (1)	20 (1)	22 (2)	20 (1)	19 (1)
Under 12	**85 (2)**	**83 (1)**	**83 (1)**	**86 (1)**	**89 (1)**	**88 (1)**	**87 (1)**	**85 (0)**
12-17	4 (1)	8 (1)	8 (1)	7 (1)	6 (1)	8 (1)	8 (1)	7 (0)
18+	10 (2)	9 (1)	10 (1)	6 (0)	6 (1)	5 (1)	6 (1)	7 (0)
12 or above	**14 (2)**	**17 (1)**	**18 (1)**	**13 (1)**	**12 (1)**	**12 (1)**	**14 (1)**	**14 (0)**
Base	*512*	*700*	*2235*	*3057*	*876*	*804*	*1590*	*9792*

* No answers and those who had never been to school are excluded from the seven age categories but included in the "All" category.

Table 4.5   CIS-R score (grouped) by educational qualifications and sex (SE in brackets)

CIS-R score	Educational qualifications*						All
	Degree	Teaching / HND, Nursing	A-level	GCSE, A–C grades or equivalent	GCSE, D–F grades or equivalent	No qualifi- cations	
	%	%	%	%	%	%	%
Women							
0-5	57 (3)	63 (2)	59 (2)	60 (1)	60 (2)	58 (1)	59 (1)
6-11	28 (2)	21 (2)	23 (2)	24 (1)	20 (2)	21 (1)	23 (1)
Under 12	**85 (2)**	**84 (2)**	**82 (2)**	**84 (1)**	**80 (2)**	**79 (1)**	**82 (1)**
12-17	8 (1)	10 (2)	11 (1)	8 (1)	9 (1)	9 (1)	9 (0)
18+	7 (1)	6 (1)	8 (1)	8 (1)	10 (2)	11 (1)	9 (1)
12 or above	**15 (2)**	**16 (2)**	**19 (2)**	**16 (1)**	**19 (2)**	**20 (1)**	**18 (1)**
Base	*450*	*463*	*442*	*1367*	*587*	*1625*	*4933*
Men							
0-5	71 (2)	76 (2)	74 (2)	74 (1)	73 (2)	71 (1)	73 (1)
6-11	18 (2)	17 (2)	14 (2)	15 (1)	17 (2)	16 (1)	16 (1)
Under 12	**89 (1)**	**93 (1)**	**89 (2)**	**89 (1)**	**90 (2)**	**87 (1)**	**89 (1)**
12-17	6 (1)	5 (1)	6 (1)	6 (1)	5 (1)	5 (1)	6 (0)
18+	4 (1)	2 (1)	6 (1)	6 (1)	5 (1)	8 (1)	6 (0)
12 or above	**10 (1)**	**7 (1)**	**12 (2)**	**12 (1)**	**10 (2)**	**13 (1)**	**12 (1)**
Base	*642*	*695*	*616*	*1174*	*474*	*1258*	*4859*
All adults							
0-5	65 (2)	70 (2)	68 (2)	66 (1)	66 (2)	64 (1)	66 (1)
6-11	22 (2)	18 (1)	17 (1)	20 (1)	19 (1)	19(1)	19 (1)
Under 12	**87 (1)**	**88 (1)**	**85 (1)**	**86 (1)**	**85 (1)**	**83 (1)**	**85 (0)**
12-17	7 (1)	7 (1)	8 (1)	7 (1)	7 (1)	7 (1)	7 (0)
18+	6 (1)	4 (1)	7 (1)	7 (1)	8 (1)	10 (1)	7 (0)
12 or above	**13 (1)**	**11 (1)**	**15 (1)**	**14 (1)**	**15 (1)**	**17 (1)**	**14 (0)**
Base	*1092*	*1157*	*1058*	*2541*	*1061*	*2883*	*9792*

* For details of educational qualifications see Glossary.

Table 4.6   CIS-R score (grouped) by employment status and sex (SE in brackets)

CIS-R score	Employment status				All
	Working full-time	Working part-time	Unemployed	Economically inactive	
	%	%	%	%	%
Women					
0-5	61 (2)	62 (1)	43 (3)	58 (1)	59 (1)
6-11	24 (1)	23 (1)	20 (2)	22 (1)	23 (1)
Under 12	**85 (1)**	**85 (1)**	**63 (3)**	**80 (1)**	**82 (1)**
12-17	9 (1)	9 (1)	14 (2)	9 (1)	9 (0)
18+	7 (1)	7 (1)	23 (3)	12 (1)	9 (1)
12 or above	**16 (1)**	**16 (1)**	**37 (3)**	**21 (1)**	**18 (1)**
Base	*1713*	*1383*	*268*	*1569*	*4933*
Men					
0-5	77 (1)	68 (3)	67 (2)	63 (2)	73 (1)
6-11	15 (1)	22 (3)	15 (2)	19 (2)	16 (1)
Under 12	**92 (1)**	**90 (2)**	**82 (2)**	**82 (2)**	**89 (1)**
12-17	5 (0)	4 (1)	9 (1)	6 (1)	6 (0)
18+	3 (0)	6 (2)	9 (1)	12 (2)	6 (0)
12 or above	**8 (1)**	**10 (2)**	**18 (2)**	**18 (2)**	**12 (1)**
Base	*3290*	*282*	*579*	*708*	*4859*
All adults					
0-5	71 (1)	63 (1)	59 (2)	59 (1)	66 (1)
6-11	18 (1)	22 (1)	17 (2)	21 (1)	19 (1)
Under 12	**89 (1)**	**85 (1)**	**76 (2)**	**80 (1)**	**85 (0)**
12-17	6 (0)	8 (1)	10 (1)	8 (1)	7 (0)
18+	4 (0)	6 (1)	13 (1)	12 (1)	7 (0)
12 or above	**10 (1)**	**14 (1)**	**23 (2)**	**20 (1)**	**14 (0)**
Base	*5003*	*1666*	*847*	*2276*	*9792*

Table 4.7   CIS-R score (grouped) by social class (based on occupation of head of family unit) and sex (SE in brackets)

CIS-R score	Social class*						All §
	I	II	IIINM	IIIM	IV	V	
	%	%	%	%	%	%	%
Women							
0-5	61 (3)	62 (2)	60 (2)	58 (2)	56 (2)	58 (3)	59 (1)
6-11	23 (2)	23 (1)	22 (1)	24 (1)	22 (1)	19 (3)	23 (1)
Under 12	**84 (2)**	**85 (1)**	**82 (1)**	**82 (1)**	**78 (2)**	**77 (3)**	**82 (1)**
12-17	9 (2)	8 (1)	8 (1)	10 (1)	11 (1)	8 (2)	9 (0)
18+	7 (1)	6 (1)	10 (1)	9 (1)	11 (1)	16 (3)	9 (1)
12 or above	**16 (2)**	**14 (1)**	**18 (1)**	**19 (1)**	**22 (2)**	**24 (3)**	**18 (1)**
Base	*285*	*1332*	*869*	*1263*	*782*	*245*	*4933*
Men							
0-5	77 (3)	71 (1)	72 (2)	74 (1)	74 (2)	73 (4)	73 (1)
6-11	17 (2)	18 (1)	15 (2)	15 (1)	16 (2)	14 (3)	16 (1)
Under 12	**94 (1)**	**89 (1)**	**87 (1)**	**89 (1)**	**90 (1)**	**87 (3)**	**89 (1)**
12-17	5 (1)	6 (1)	6 (1)	5 (1)	6 (1)	5 (1)	6 (0)
18+	1 (2)	5 (6)	7 (1)	6 (1)	5 (1)	8 (2)	5 (0)
12 or above	**6 (1)**	**11 (1)**	**13 (1)**	**11 (1)**	**11 (1)**	**13 (3)**	**11 (1)**
Base	*364*	*1222*	*614*	*1514*	*700*	*266*	*4859*
All adults							
0-5	70 (2)	66 (1)	65 (2)	67 (1)	64 (1)	66 (2)	66 (1)
6-11	20 (2)	20 (1)	19 (1)	19 (1)	19 (1)	16 (2)	19 (1)
Under 12	**90 (1)**	**86 (1)**	**84 (1)**	**86 (1)**	**84 (1)**	**82 (2)**	**85 (0)**
12-17	6 (1)	7 (1)	8 (1)	7 (1)	8 (1)	6 (1)	7 (0)
18+	4 (1)	6 (1)	8 (1)	7 (1)	8 (1)	12 (2)	7 (0)
12 or above	**10 (1)**	**13 (1)**	**16 (1)**	**14 (1)**	**16 (1)**	**18 (2)**	**14 (0)**
Base	*649*	*2554*	*1484*	*2776*	*1482*	*511*	*9792*

* I = Professional; II = Employers and Managers; IIINM = Intermediate and Junior Non-Manual; IIIM = Skilled manual and own account non-professional; IV = Semi-skilled Manual and Personal service;   V = Unskilled manual.

§ No answers, members of the Armed Forces, full-time students and those who have never worked are excluded from the six social class categories but included in the "All" category.

Table 4.8   CIS-R score (grouped) by family unit type and sex (SE in brackets)

CIS-R score	Family unit type*						All
	Couple, no child	Couple & child(ren)	Lone parent & child(ren)	One person only	Adult with parents	Adult with one parent	
	%	%	%	%	%	%	%
Women							
0-5	64 (2)	59 (1)	50 (2)	52 (2)	66 (3)	55 (6)	59 (1)
6-11	22 (1)	23 (1)	23 (2)	25 (2)	22 (3)	28 (5)	23 (1)
Under 12	**86 (1)**	**82 (1)**	**72 (2)**	**77 (2)**	**88 (2)**	**83 (4)**	**82 (1)**
12-17	8 (1)	9 (1)	12 (1)	10 (1)	4 (1)	12 (3)	9 (0)
18+	6 (1)	8 (1)	15 (1)	13 (1)	8 (2)	5 (3)	9 (1)
12 or above	**14 (1)**	**18 (1)**	**28 (2)**	**23 (2)**	**12 (2)**	**17 (4)**	**18 (1)**
Base	*1342*	*1957*	*502*	*593*	*424*	*115*	*4933*
Men							
0-5	75 (1)	73 (1)	63 (6)	67 (2)	77 (2)	71 (4)	73 (1)
6-11	15 (1)	16 (1)	17 (4)	16 (2)	16 (2)	16 (3)	16 (1)
Under 12	**90 (1)**	**89 (1)**	**80 (5)**	**84 (1)**	**93 (1)**	**87 (3)**	**89 (0)**
12-17	4 (1)	5 (1)	11 (4)	9 (1)	3 (1)	10 (3)	6 (0)
18+	5 (1)	6 (1)	9 (3)	7 (1)	4 (1)	3 (1)	6 (0)
12 or above	**10 (1)**	**11 (1)**	**20 (5)**	**16 (1)**	**7 (1)**	**13 (3)**	**11 (0)**
Base	*1237*	*1974*	*63*	*724*	*664*	*198*	*4859*
All adults							
0-5	69 (1)	66 (1)	51 (2)	60 (1)	73 (2)	65 (3)	66 (1)
6-11	18 (1)	20 (1)	22 (2)	20 (1)	18 (2)	21 (3)	19 (1)
Under 12	**88 (1)**	**84 (1)**	**73 (2)**	**81 (1)**	**91 (1)**	**76 (2)**	**85 (0)**
12-17	6 (1)	7 (0)	12 (1)	10 (1)	4 (1)	10 (2)	7 (0)
18+	6 (1)	7 (0)	15 (1)	10 (1)	5 (1)	4 (1)	7 (0)
12 or above	**12 (1)**	**14 (1)**	**27 (2)**	**19 (1)**	**9 (1)**	**14 (2)**	**15 (0)**
Base	*2578*	*3931*	*564*	*1317*	*1088*	*313*	*9792*

* For details of family unit type, see Glossary.

Table 4.9 CIS-R score (grouped) by tenure and sex (SE in brackets)

CIS-R score	Tenure				All
	Owned outright	Owned with mortgage	Rented from LA or HA	Rented from other source	
	%	%	%	%	%
Women					
0-5	68 (2)	61 (1)	50 (2)	52 (3)	59 (1)
6-11	19 (1)	23 (1)	24 (1)	28 (2)	23 (1)
Under 12	**87 (1)**	**84 (1)**	**74 (2)**	**79 (2)**	**82 (1)**
12-17	8 (1)	8 (1)	11 (1)	11 (1)	9 (0)
18+	6 (1)	8 (1)	14 (1)	10 (2)	9 (1)
12 or above	**14 (1)**	**16 (1)**	**25 (2)**	**21 (2)**	**18 (1)**
Base	*842*	*2659*	*1008*	*424*	*4933*
Men					
0-5	80 (2)	75 (1)	64 (2)	66 (2)	73 (1)
6-11	12 (1)	16 (1)	18 (1)	20 (2)	16 (1)
Under 12	**92 (1)**	**91 (1)**	**82 (1)**	**86 (2)**	**89 (1)**
12-17	4 (1)	5 (0)	8 (1)	8 (1)	6 (0)
18+	4 (1)	5 (0)	10 (1)	7 (1)	6 (0)
12 or above	**8 (1)**	**10 (1)**	**18 (1)**	**14 (2)**	**12 (1)**
Base	*752*	*2834*	*792*	*481*	*4859*
All adults					
0-5	73 (1)	68 (1)	56 (1)	59 (2)	66 (1)
6-11	16 (1)	19 (1)	21 (1)	23 (1)	19 (1)
Under 12	**89 (1)**	**87 (1)**	**78 (1)**	**82 (1)**	**85 (0)**
12-17	6 (1)	6 (0)	10 (1)	9 (1)	7 (0)
18+	5 (1)	6 (0)	12 (1)	8 (1)	7 (0)
12 or above	**11 (1)**	**12 (1)**	**22 (1)**	**17 (1)**	**14 (0)**
Base	*1595*	*5493*	*1800*	*905*	*9792*

Table 4.10   CIS-R score (grouped) by type of accommodation and sex (SE in brackets)

CIS-R score	Type of accommodation				All
	Detached	Semi-detached	Terraced	Flat or maisonette	
	%	%	%	%	%
Women					
0-5	64 (2)	63 (2)	56 (1)	51 (2)	59 (1)
6-11	21 (1)	22 (1)	23 (1)	25 (2)	23 (1)
Under 12	**85 (1)**	**84 (1)**	**79 (1)**	**76 (2)**	**82 (1)**
12-17	8 (1)	8 (1)	10 (1)	10 (1)	9 (0)
18+	6 (1)	8 (1)	11 (1)	13 (1)	9 (1)
12 or above	**14 (1)**	**16 (1)**	**21 (1)**	**23 (2)**	**18 (1)**
Base	*1075*	*1582*	*1518*	*758*	*4933*
Men					
0-5	75 (2)	76 (1)	72 (1)	66 (2)	73 (1)
6-11	16 (2)	14 (1)	16 (1)	18 (2)	16 (1)
Under 12	**91 (1)**	**90 (1)**	**88 (1)**	**84 (1)**	**89 (1)**
12-17	5 (1)	5 (1)	6 (1)	8 (1)	6 (0)
18+	4 (1)	5 (1)	6 (1)	8 (1)	6 (0)
12 or above	**9 (1)**	**10 (1)**	**12 (1)**	**16 (1)**	**12 (1)**
Base	*1038*	*1679*	*1441*	*701*	*4859*
All adults					
0-5	70 (1)	70 (1)	64 (1)	58 (2)	66 (1)
6-11	19 (1)	18 (1)	20 (1)	22 (1)	19 (1)
Under 12	**89 (1)**	**88 (1)**	**84 (1)**	**80 (1)**	**85 (0)**
12-17	6 (1)	6 (0)	8 (1)	9 (1)	7 (0)
18+	5 (1)	6 (1)	8 (1)	11 (1)	7 (0)
12 or above	**11 (1)**	**13 (1)**	**16 (1)**	**20 (1)**	**14 (0)**
Base	*2113*	*3261*	*2960*	*1458*	*9792*

25

Table 4.11   CIS-R score (grouped) by ownership of van or car and sex (SE in brackets)

CIS-R score	Ownership of van or car				All
	No car or van	1 car or van	2 cars or vans	3 or more cars or vans	
	%	%	%	%	%
Women					
0-5	51 (2)	59 (1)	64 (2)	63 (3)	59 (1)
6-11	24 (1)	22 (1)	22 (1)	25 (3)	23 (1)
Under 12	**75 (1)**	**81 (1)**	**86 (1)**	**88 (2)**	**82 (1)**
12-17	10 (1)	10 (1)	8 (1)	9 (2)	9 (0)
18+	16 (1)	9 (1)	6 (1)	3 (1)	9 (1)
12 or above	**26 (1)**	**19 (1)**	**14 (1)**	**12 (2)**	**18 (1)**
Base	*980*	*2220*	*1403*	*330*	*4933*
Men					
0-5	63 (2)	73 (1)	76 (1)	80 (2)	73 (1)
6-11	18 (1)	16 (1)	16 (1)	12 (2)	16 (1)
Under 12	**81 (1)**	**89 (1)**	**92 (1)**	**92 (1)**	**89 (1)**
12-17	8 (1)	6 (1)	4 (1)	4 (1)	6 (0)
18+	10 (1)	5 (0)	4 (1)	5 (1)	6 (0)
12 or above	**18 (1)**	**11 (1)**	**8 (1)**	**9 (1)**	**12 (1)**
Base	*749*	*2240*	*1443*	*426*	*4859*
All adults					
0-5	56 (1)	66 (1)	70 (1)	72 (2)	66 (1)
6-11	21 (1)	19 (1)	19 (1)	18 (2)	19 (1)
Under 12	**77 (1)**	**85 (1)**	**89 (1)**	**90 (1)**	**85 (0)**
12-17	9 (1)	8 (0)	6 (1)	6 (1)	7 (0)
18+	13 (1)	7 (0)	5 (1)	4 (1)	7 (0)
12 or above	**22 (1)**	**15 (1)**	**11 (1)**	**10 (1)**	**14 (0)**
Base	*1729*	*4461*	*2846*	*756*	*9792*

Table 4.12 Proportion of adults with an overall score of 12 or more on each CIS-R symptom by type of accommodation, tenure, marital status, employment status and sex

	Living in detached or semi-detached house				Living in terraced house, maisonette or flat			
	Bought outright/ mortgage		Rented from LA, HA, other		Bought outright/ mortgage		Rented from LA, HA, other	
	Proportion with CIS-R score of 12 or more	*Base*	Proportion with CIS-R score of 12 or more	*Base*	Proportion with CIS-R score of 12 or more	*Base*	Proportion with CIS-R score of 12 or more	*Base*
Women								
Married and working	13	*(1155)*	15	*(133)*	16	*(623)*	20	*(225)*
Single, widowed, divorced, separated and working	13	*(368)*	16	*(87)*	20	*(288)*	19	*(207)*
Married and not working	14	*(522)*	22	*(133)*	21	*(264)*	31	*(233)*
Single, widowed, divorced, separated and not working	24	*(149)*	23	*(99)*	22	*(121)*	34	*(309)*
Men								
Married and working	7	*(1403)*	11	*(171)*	8	*(711)*	12	*(231)*
Single, widowed, divorced, separated and working	5	*(425)*	12	*(103)*	10	*(309)*	15	*(204)*
Married and not working	13	*(264)*	23	*(88)*	22	*(165)*	21	*(163)*
Single, widowed, divorced, separated and not working	14	*(174)*	19	*(77)*	13	*(121)*	22	*(223)*

27

Table 4.13 CIS-R score (grouped) by Regional Health Authority (RHA) and sex (SE in brackets)

CIS-R score	RHA								
	Northern	Yorkshire	Trent	East Anglia	NW Thames	NE Thames	SE Thames	SW Thames	Wessex
	%	%	%	%	%	%	%	%	%
Women									
0-5	58 (3)	54 (4)	68 (2)	60 (5)	60 (4)	48 (4)	50 (2)	56 (5)	66 (5)
6-11	24 (3)	26 (3)	20 (2)	24 (1)	21 (2)	26 (3)	29 (3)	24 (3)	21 (3)
Under 12	**82 (3)**	**80 (3)**	**88 (2)**	**84 (4)**	**81 (3)**	**74 (2)**	**79 (3)**	**80 (4)**	**87 (3)**
12-17	8 (2)	11 (2)	7 (1)	10 (1)	11 (2)	12 (2)	12 (2)	12 (2)	7 (3)
18+	10 (2)	9 (2)	5 (1)	7 (3)	8 (1)	14 (2)	9 (2)	8 (3)	7 (1)
12 or above	**18 (3)**	**20 (3)**	**12 (2)**	**17 (4)**	**19 (3)**	**26 (2)**	**21 (3)**	**20 (4)**	**14 (3)**
Base	*262*	*352*	*429*	*207*	*318*	*308*	*354*	*255*	*299*
Men									
0-5	74 (3)	75 (2)	72 (3)	78 (6)	71 (4)	70 (5)	73 (3)	71 (3)	76 (3)
6-11	12 (2)	15 (2)	17 (2)	16 (5)	18 (3)	18 (4)	17 (3)	18 (3)	14 (2)
Under 12	**86 (2)**	**90 (1)**	**89 (2)**	**94 (2)**	**89 (2)**	**88 (2)**	**90 (2)**	**89 (2)**	**90 (2)**
12-17	7 (2)	4 (1)	5 (1)	4 (2)	4 (1)	6 (1)	5 (1)	7 (2)	6 (2)
18+	6 (2)	6 (1)	6 (1)	2 (1)	7 (1)	7 (1)	5 (2)	4 (1)	4 (1)
12 or above	**13 (2)**	**10 (1)**	**11 (2)**	**6 (2)**	**11 (2)**	**13 (2)**	**10 (2)**	**11 (2)**	**10 (2)**
Base	*265*	*331*	*498*	*173*	*327*	*325*	*327*	*269*	*294*
All adults									
0-5	66 (2)	64 (2)	70 (2)	68 (5)	66 (4)	59 (4)	61 (3)	64 (3)	71 (4)
6-11	18 (1)	20 (2)	18 (1)	20 (3)	20 (2)	22 (3)	23 (3)	21 (3)	17 (3)
Under 12	**84 (2)**	**84 (2)**	**88 (1)**	**88 (3)**	**86 (2)**	**81 (2)**	**84 (2)**	**85 (2)**	**88 (2)**
12-17	7 (1)	7 (1)	6 (1)	7 (1)	8 (1)	9 (1)	9 (1)	9 (1)	7 (2)
18+	8 (1)	8 (1)	5 (1)	4 (2)	7 (1)	10 (1)	7 (1)	6 (2)	5 (1)
12 or above	**15 (2)**	**15 (2)**	**11 (1)**	**11 (3)**	**15 (2)**	**19 (2)**	**16 (2)**	**15 (2)**	**12 (2)**
Base	*527*	*683*	*927*	*380*	*644*	*634*	*680*	*524*	*594*

								All	
Oxford	South Western	West Midlands	Mersey	North Western	England	Scotland	Wales		
%	%	%	%	%	%	%	%	%	
									Women
70 (5)	64 (3)	57 (4)	54 (2)	64 (3)	59 (1)	61 (3)	57 (4)	59 (1)	0-5
15 (2)	23 (2)	24 (3)	23 (1)	19 (3)	23 (1)	22 (2)	22 (4)	23 (1)	6-11
85 (3)	**87 (1)**	**81 (2)**	**77 (3)**	**83 (2)**	**81 (1)**	**83 (3)**	**80 (3)**	**82 (1)**	**Under 12**
8 (3)	6 (2)	9 (2)	11 (3)	7 (1)	9 (1)	8 (2)	7 (2)	9 (0)	12-17
6 (1)	7 (2)	10 (2)	13 (2)	11 (2)	9 (1)	10 (2)	14 (4)	9 (1)	18+
14 (3)	**13 (1)**	**19 (2)**	**24 (3)**	**18 (2)**	**18 (1)**	**18 (3)**	**21 (3)**	**18 (1)**	**12 or above**
243	*259*	*434*	*234*	*362*	*4317*	*362*	*254*	*4933*	*Base*
									Men
76 (5)	73 (3)	71 (2)	68 (3)	74 (3)	73 (1)	75 (3)	72 (4)	73 (1)	0-5
14 (3)	18 (3)	15 (2)	19 (3)	15 (2)	16 (1)	15 (2)	16 (4)	16 (1)	6-11
90 (3)	**91 (2)**	**85 (1)**	**87 (3)**	**89 (2)**	**89 (1)**	**90 (2)**	**88 (3)**	**89 (1)**	**Under 12**
6 (2)	6 (1)	6 (1)	7 (2)	4 (1)	5 (0)	5 (1)	7 (1)	6 (0)	12-17
5 (2)	2 (1)	8 (1)	6 (1)	6 (1)	6 (0)	6 (1)	6 (1)	6 (0)	18+
11 (3)	**8 (2)**	**14 (1)**	**13 (3)**	**10 (2)**	**11 (1)**	**11 (2)**	**11 (3)**	**12 (1)**	**12 or above**
259	*261*	*429*	*200*	*339*	*4297*	*316*	*245*	*4859*	*Base*
									All adults
73 (5)	69 (2)	64 (2)	60 (1)	69 (3)	66 (1)	67 (2)	65 (2)	66 (1)	0-5
14 (2)	21 (2)	20 (2)	21 (2)	17 (2)	20 (1)	18 (1)	19 (2)	19 (1)	6-11
87 (3)	**90 (1)**	**84 (1)**	**81 (2)**	**86 (2)**	**86 (0)**	**85 (2)**	**84 (2)**	**85 (0)**	**Under 12**
7 (2)	6 (1)	7 (1)	9 (2)	6 (1)	7 (0)	6 (1)	7 (2)	7 (0)	12-17
6 (2)	5 (1)	9 (1)	9 (1)	8 (1)	7 (0)	8 (1)	9 (2)	7 (0)	18+
13 (3)	**11 (1)**	**16 (1)**	**18 (2)**	**14 (2)**	**14 (0)**	**14 (2)**	**16 (2)**	**14 (0)**	**12 or above**
502	*520*	*863*	*434*	*701*	*8614*	*678*	*499*	*9792*	*Base*

Table 4.14   CIS-R score (grouped) by locality and sex (SE in brackets)

CIS-R score	Locality			All
	Urban	Semi-rural	Rural	
	%	%	%	%
Women				
0-5	57 (1)	63 (2)	66 (3)	59 (1)
6-11	23 (1)	22 (1)	20 (2)	23 (1)
Under 12	**80 (1)**	**85 (1)**	**86 (2)**	**82 (1)**
12-17	10 (1)	7 (1)	8 (2)	9 (0)
18+	10 (1)	7 (1)	6 (1)	9 (1)
12 or above	**20 (1)**	**14 (1)**	**14 (2)**	**18 (1)**
Base	*3263*	*1179*	*492*	*4933*
Men				
0-5	72 (1)	74 (1)	78 (2)	73 (1)
6-11	16 (1)	16 (1)	16 (1)	16 (1)
Under 12	**88 (1)**	**90 (1)**	**94 (1)**	**89 (1)**
12-17	6 (1)	6 (1)	4 (1)	6 (0)
18+	6 (0)	5 (1)	2 (1)	6 (0)
12 or above	**12 (1)**	**11 (1)**	**6 (1)**	**12 (1)**
Base	*3187*	*1153*	*519*	*4859*
All adults				
0-5	64 (1)	69 (1)	72 (2)	66 (1)
6-11	20 (1)	19 (1)	18 (1)	19 (1)
Under 12	**84 (1)**	**88 (1)**	**90 (1)**	**85 (0)**
12-17	8 (0)	6 (1)	6 (1)	7 (0)
18+	8 (0)	6 (1)	4 (1)	7 (0)
12 or above	**16 (1)**	**12 (1)**	**10 (1)**	**14 (0)**
Base	*6450*	*2332*	*1010*	*9792*

Table 4.15 Odds ratios of socio-demographic correlates of CIS-R score

CIS-R score of 12 or more		Adjusted OR	(95% CI)
Sex	Male	1.00	....
	Female	1.56**	(1.37-1.78)
Age	16-24	1.00	....
	25-34	1.07	(0.87-1.32)
	35-44	1.23	(0.99-1.53)
	45-54	1.24	(0.99-1.55)
	55-64	0.72**	(0.56-0.91)
Family unit type	Couple, no children	1.00	....
	Couple: 1+ child	1.03	(0.87-1.21)
	Lone parent + child	1.56**	(1.26-1.93)
	One person only	1.48**	(1.25-1.76)
	Adult with parents	0.76	(0.54-1.05)
	Adult with one parent	0.80	(0.54-1.19)
Employment status	Working full time	1.00	....
	Working part time	1.19	(1.00-1.42)
	Unemployed	2.26**	(1.87-2.72)
	Economically inactive	1.71**	(1.47-2.00)
Accommodation	Detached	1.00	
	Semi-detached	0.96	(0.80-1.15)
	Terraced	1.19	(1.00-1.43)
	Flat/maisonette	1.15	(0.93-1.43)
Tenure	Owner/occupier	1.00	....
	Renter	1.33**	(1.16-1.53)
Locality	Semi-rural/rural	1.00	....
	Urban	1.21**	(1.06-1.38)

Significance: *   p<0.05

           ** p<0.01

5 Prevalence of neurotic symptoms

5.1 Introduction

This chapter looks at the fourteen neurotic symptoms covered by the Revised Clinical Interview Schedule (CIS-R), and how they related to personal, family and household characteristics, region and locality. As well as presenting the prevalence of neurotic symptoms, odds ratios are shown which summarise the effects of the socio-demographic variables on the odds of having each symptom.

The fourteen symptoms covered by the CIS-R are:

> Fatigue
> Sleep problems
> Irritability
> Worry (excluding worry about physical health)
> Depression
> Depressive ideas
> Anxiety
> Obsessions
> Concentration and forgetfulness
> Somatic symptoms
> Compulsions
> Phobias
> Worry about physical health
> Panic

In this chapter terms such as depression, anxiety and phobias refer to the symptoms as they are rated by the CIS-R.

Because the symptoms are not mutually exclusive, informants may have had multiple symptoms.

Symptom scores

Informants were rated on all fourteen symptoms. For each symptom they were assigned scores of between 0 and 4 depending on whether the symptom was present in the past week, and on various measures of the frequency, duration and severity of the symptom. This chapter reports on symptoms of moderate to high severity which were experienced in the past week, that is, where the symptom score was two or more (see section 2.1 and Appendix B).

Four symptoms stood out as most common among both men and women. These were fatigue, sleep problems, irritability and worry (not including worry about physical health). The proportions of all adults experiencing these symptoms in the week before interview were between 27%, for fatigue, and 20% for worry. The next most frequently occurring symptoms were depression, depressive ideas, anxiety and obsessions (each affecting about 10% of respondents). Panic had the lowest prevalence, 2%. (*Figure 5.1*)

5.2 Distribution of neurotic symptoms by personal characteristics

Sex

Women were considerably more likely to have each neurotic symptom than men. They were around twice as likely to have somatic symptoms and phobias, and over one and a half times more likely to suffer fatigue, obsessions, poor concentration and forgetfulness, compulsions and depressive ideas. Because differences between men and women were statistically significant for all symptoms except worry about physical health, all prevalence tables are presented separately for women, men and then for all adults. (*Figure 5.2*)

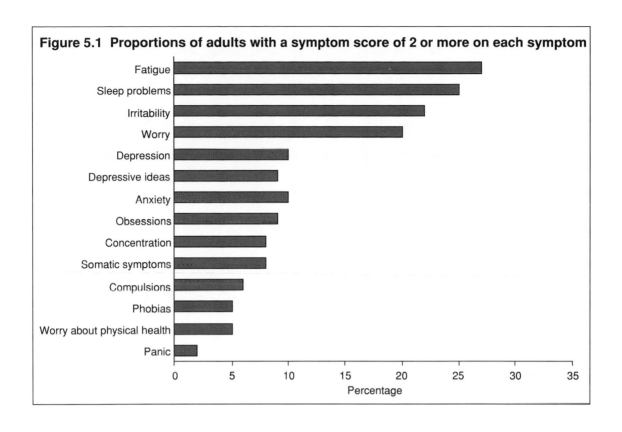

Figure 5.1 Proportions of adults with a symptom score of 2 or more on each symptom

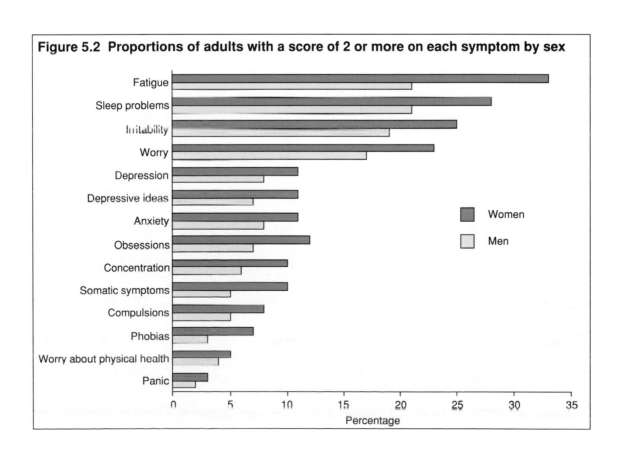

Figure 5.2 Proportions of adults with a score of 2 or more on each symptom by sex

Age

There were few pronounced differences in the experience of neurotic symptoms with age. The only symptom which showed a marked relationship with age was irritability among women, which declined with increasing age. Compared with women overall, those aged 55 to 64 years were half as likely to have felt irritable or have had depressive ideas. Men aged 16 to 19 years differed from men overall, having the smallest proportions who suffered fatigue, worry, somatic symptoms and worry about physical health. *(Table 5.1)*

Ethnicity

Because only 4% of the sample regarded themselves as West Indian, African, Asian or Oriental, any apparent differences in the prevalence of symptoms between ethnic groups are difficult to interpret.

In general, differences between women according to their ethnic group were small, with a few notable exceptions. Compared with White women, depression appeared to be twice as prevalent among West Indian and African women, and Asian and Oriental women; this was a statistically significant finding only for West Indian and African women. Also compared with White women, Asian and Oriental women were over three times as likely to worry about their physical health (significant) and West Indian and African women appeared twice as likely to have compulsions (not significant).

Asian and Oriental men appeared less likely than White men to have a number of symptoms, notably fatigue and compulsions (both significant), and irritability. Several neurotic symptoms appeared to be more prevalent among West Indian and African men than their White counterparts; differences in the prevalence of depressive ideas and worry about physical health were more than two-fold. However, these results should be treated with caution. Owing to the small number of West Indian and African men studied, none of the differences observed between this group and White men reached statistical significance.

Marital status

The prevalence of many symptoms varied considerably among women according to their marital status. Most neurotic symptoms were least prevalent among married women and most prevalent among divorced women. There was no clear pattern for those who were cohabiting, single, or widowed. In comparison with married women, a number of symptoms seemed to be more prevalent among separated women.

Among men the lowest prevalence rates of neurotic symptoms were generally found among those who were married, cohabiting or single. Although the number of separated men was small, they were notable for having significantly higher prevalence of many symptoms compared with married, cohabiting and single men. *(Table 5.3)*

Education

No clear relationship was found between the prevalence of symptoms and either the age at which informants finished their full-time education or the highest educational qualification they attained. *(Tables 5.4 and 5.5)*

Employment status

There was a strong association between people's employment status and neurotic symptoms. Almost all symptoms were considerably more prevalent among unemployed women compared with those who worked full-time and differences in prevalence were more than two-fold for a number of symptoms: depression, depressive ideas, anxiety, obsessions, poor concentration and forgetfulness and phobias. Economically inactive women were also more likely to have a number of symptoms than those who were working full time, notably; sleep problems, depression, depressive ideas, phobias and worry about physical health.

For men, the highest prevalence of neurotic symptoms was among those who were economically inactive. Compared with men who worked full time, economically inactive men were more likely to have each symptom except irritability, worry and phobias; for most symptoms the differences were more than two-fold. The prevalence rates of most symptoms were also higher among unemployed men than among those working full time but the differences were not as great as for economically inactive men.*(Table 5.6)*

5.3 Distribution of neurotic symptoms by family and household characteristics

Social class

The prevalence of neurotic symptoms varied with social class in the same way as the overall CIS-R score (section 4.2). Women in social classes I and II (Professionals, and Employers and Managers) appeared less likely than others to have almost every symptom, although these differences were not statistically significant (Figure 5.3). Among men, only those in social class I (Professionals) appeared less likely than others to have each neurotic symptom. *(Table 5.7 and Figure 5.3)*

Family unit type

The greatest variations in the prevalence of symptoms by the type of family unit were observed among women. Compared with married and cohabiting women, lone mothers and women in one-person family units[1], appeared more likely to have each symptom. In particular, lone mothers had higher rates of all symptoms except for fatigue, worry about physical health and panic compared with married women with children.

For married women, having children appeared to increase the likelihood of having a number of symptoms; most notably, those with children were one and a half times more likely to suffer irritability than those without children. Indeed, irritability appears to be related to having children; it was also one and a half times more

prevalent among lone mothers than among single women.

Similar patterns were found for men, although the magnitude of variations was smaller and there were very few lone fathers. *(Table 5.8)*

Tenure

Owner-occupiers were much less likely to have neurotic symptoms than adults who rented their homes. Differences were particularly marked between adults who rented from a local authority (LA) or a housing association (HA) and those who owned their homes outright without a mortgage. Compared with women who owned their homes outright, women who rented from an LA or HA were more than twice as likely to have depression, depressive ideas, anxiety and panic. The same comparison among men showed that those who rented from an LA or HA were more than twice as likely to have experienced worry, depressive ideas, poor concentration and forgetfulness, somatic symptoms, compulsions, phobias and panic. Depressive ideas were around three times more prevalent among LA and HA renters than among those who owned their homes outright.

Renters in the private sector were also more likely to have each neurotic symptom than owners. Although these differences were large, especially among men, they were not as great as for LA or HA renters. *(Table 5.9)*

Type of accommodation

For men and women, the highest prevalence of almost every symptom was found among those living in flats or maisonettes. Differences between adults living in flats or maisonettes and those in detached homes were two-fold or greater for a number of symptoms although not all differences were statistically significant. Among women, living in a terraced home was also associated with increased prevalence of some symptoms compared with living in a detached home. *(Table 5.10)*

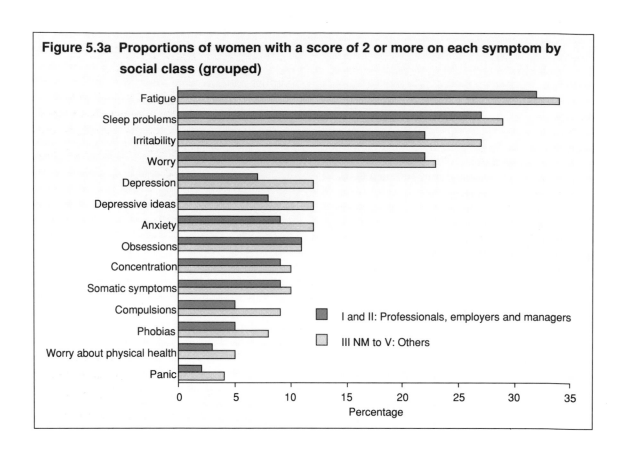

Figure 5.3a Proportions of women with a score of 2 or more on each symptom by social class (grouped)

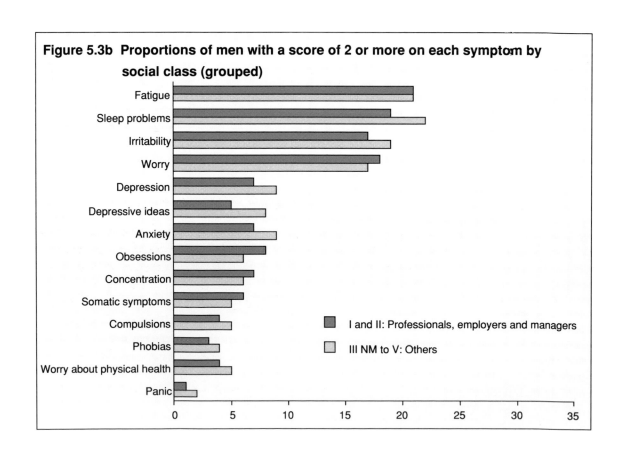

Figure 5.3b Proportions of men with a score of 2 or more on each symptom by social class (grouped)

5.4 Distribution of neurotic symptoms by region and locality

Country and region

There was little variation in the prevalence of neurotic symptoms between the 14 Regional Health Authorities of England, and Scotland and Wales.[2]

Although differences were not generally marked, some RHAs tended to have the lowest proportions of adults with any symptoms while other RHAs tended to have the highest proportions. Men in East Anglia RHA and women in Oxford RHA had low rates for many symptoms but men in East Anglia RHA were less likely to be unemployed or economically inactive than others, and women in Oxford RHA were less likely than other to be economically inactive or lone mothers. A number of RHAs tended to have the highest rates for many symptoms, in particular North East Thames. Most of these RHAs were characterised by high rates of unemployment and economic inactivity, and high proportions of lone parents.

RHAs which showed significantly higher prevalence of symptoms than the national average for women were South East Thames with respect to worry and North East Thames (anxiety and somatic symptoms). RHAs with below average rates for women on any symptoms were Oxford with respect to somatic symptoms, South Western (compulsions) and East Anglia (worry about physical health). Men in East Anglia RHA had lower than average rates of depressive ideas, poor concentration and forgetfulness and somatic symptoms. There were also lower than average rates for men in the South Western RHA for anxiety, and men in North West RHA for obsessions.

However, multi-variate analysis shows that once other factors are considered, there was no significant association between Regional Health Authority and neurotic symptoms.
(Table 5.11)

Locality

For both men and women, neurotic symptoms were most prevalent in urban areas and least prevalent in rural areas. Furthermore, for many symptoms the prevalence among women in urban areas was higher than among those in semi-rural areas. However, because the number of men in rural areas was small, most of the differences observed between men in urban and rural areas did not reach statistical significance. *(Table 5.12)*

5.5 Odds ratios of socio-demographic correlates of neurotic symptoms

Multiple logistic regression was used to produce odds ratios for the socio-demographic correlates of each of the fourteen symptoms.[3] The odds ratios produced show the increase or decrease in the likelihood that an individual in a particular group had a symptom compared with an individual in a reference group (for which the odds ratio is 1.00) while taking into account the possible confounding effects of other socio-demographic variables. All the socio-demographic variables which were considered earlier were entered into the logistic regression model: sex, age, ethnicity, marital status, age finished full-time education, educational level, employment status, social class, family unit type, tenure, type of accommodation, region and locality.

The odds ratios are summarised in Table 5.13 and are presented for each symptom with confidence intervals in Tables 5.14 to 5.27. The summary table shows the population subgroups for which the odds of having the symptoms were significantly different from the reference group at the 5% level.

Four socio-demographic correlates had the most wide-ranging effects in that they were associated with almost all of the 14 symptoms. These were sex, employment status, family unit type, and tenure.

37

Sex was a highly significant correlate of all symptoms except depression and worry about physical health; employment status was correlated with all except fatigue; and tenure with all but obsessions and somatic symptoms. The type of family unit was correlated with all symptoms although the correlations between symptoms and the various types of family unit were quite complex.

In general, in terms of the magnitude of these correlations, the single factor with the greatest association with the prevalence of a symptom was employment status, and in particular whether the person was unemployed or economically inactive rather than working full time (odds ratios for the unemployed and economically inactive were in the range 1.20 to 2.66). Sex had the next greatest association (odds ratios for women were in the range 1.31 to 2.07), followed by the type of family unit (odds ratios across all categories ranged from 1.18 to 1.78 and 0.37 to 0.84) and tenure (odds ratios for renters ranged from 1.16 to 1.43).

The results of the multivariate analyses for each socio-demographic variable that was included in the model are reported below. The four variables which were most highly correlated with neurotic symptoms are presented first: sex, employment status, family unit type and tenure. *(Tables 5.13 to 5.27)*

Sex

As the summary table shows, sex was a highly significant correlate of all symptoms except depression and worry about physical health, with women more likely to have any of the symptoms than men. Women had more than twice the odds of having phobic symptoms than men (odds ratio=2.07) and over one and a half times the odds of having fatigue (OR=1.76), depressive ideas (OR=1.53), obsessions (OR=1.64), somatic symptoms (OR=1.74) and panic (OR=1.74).

Employment status

Employment status was very highly correlated with all symptoms, except fatigue. Of all factors which were studied, being unemployed made the single greatest difference to the odds of having these symptoms. After controlling for the other factors, unemployed adults had around twice the odds of having sleep problems, depression, anxiety, phobias, worry about physical health, and panic compared with people who were working full time (OR between 1.85 to 2.14) and had over two and a half times the odds of experiencing depressive ideas and obsessions (OR=2.66 and 2.51 respectively).

Economic inactivity was also associated with significantly increased odds of having all symptoms except fatigue, although the associations were generally not as pronounced as among the unemployed. Compared with full-time workers economically inactive informants had between one and a half and two times the odds of having sleep problems, depression and depressive ideas, anxiety, obsessions, concentration and forgetfulness, somatic symptoms and phobia (OR between 1.50 and 2.00). They had more then twice the odds of worrying about their physical health (OR=2.58) and panic (OR=2.21).

Working part time rather than full time made little significant difference to the odds of having the symptoms. However, part-time workers were around 20% to 40% more likely to have experienced sleep problems, depressive ideas, obsessions and compulsions than those working full time (OR around 1.20 to 1.40).

Family unit type

Although being in some types of family unit types significantly increased or decreased the odds of having some symptoms, there was not a clear pattern. The reference group was married (or cohabiting) adults with no children. Compared to people in the reference group, being married with children increased the odds of having irritability (OR=1.37) but decreased the odds of having sleep problems, obsessions, compulsions and worry about physical health by between 20% and 30% (OR between 0.70 and 0.80).

Being a lone parent increased the odds of having fatigue, irritability, depression, obsessions, concentration problems and forgetfulness and somatic symptoms compared with being married without children by about 25% to 45%, and the odds of having depressive ideas were over 75% higher than among the reference group (OR=1.78).

People in a 'one-person family unit', mostly people who lived alone[1], had increased odds of having fatigue, sleep problems, worry, depression, depressive ideas, anxiety, obsessions, concentration problems and forgetfulness, somatic symptoms and phobias (OR between 1.18 and 1.80), compared with those in the reference group, but the odds of having irritability were lower (0.84).

Adults who were living with both parents showed lower odds of sleep problems, obsessions, somatic symptoms and worry about physical health compared with the reference group (OR between 0.37 and 0.64). Adults who lived with a lone parent were about 45% less likely to have fatigue and around 50% less likely to suffer somatic symptoms.

Tenure

People who lived in rented accommodation were significantly more likely to have all symptoms except obsessions and somatic symptoms compared with people who were owner-occupiers; for most symptoms the odds among renters of having the symptom were up to 45% higher. Renting increased the odds of experiencing panic almost two-fold (OR=1.95).

Age

Lower odds of irritability, worry, depression, depressive ideas, obsession, compulsions and phobias were found among older age groups. Compared with the 16 to 24 years reference group, the odds of having irritability among 35

to 44 year olds were 25% lower, and for 45 to 54 year olds and 55 to 64 year olds they were 45% and 65% lower respectively. Also adults aged 45 to 64 had lower odds of compulsions and phobias than 16 to 24 year olds by about 30% to 50%.

Compared with 16 to 24 year olds, adults aged 35 to 44 years and 45 to 54 years had considerably higher odds of having anxiety (by 60% to 90%) and somatic symptoms (by 40% to 70%), and 35 to 44 year olds were more likely to worry about their physical health.

Ethnicity

Allowing for other factors, differences between ethnic groups were found for three symptoms: irritability, depression and worry about physical health. Asian and Oriental adults were about 45% less likely than Whites to have irritability (OR=0.56) but almost twice as likely to worry about their physical health (OR=1.94). West Indian and African adults were almost 70% more likely than Whites to have depression (OR=1.67).

Education

Having no qualifications or qualifications below GCE 'O' level standard increased the odds of having three symptoms, depression, phobias and worry about physical health by around 40% to 50% in comparison with adults who had GCE 'A' level or equivalent, or higher qualifications.

The age at which informants finished their full-time education was not identified as a significant correlate of neurotic symptoms when all other factors were considered.

Social class

Whether the informants were in a manual or non-manual social class was also identified as a factor for which differences in the odds of having symptoms were significant. Adults in manual social classes were more likely to suffer depressive ideas (OR=1.17) and compulsions

(OR=1.26) than those in non-manual social classes.

Type of accommodation

People living in terraced houses had 20% lower odds of having worry but 60% higher odds of having worry about physical health compared with those living in a detached property. People living in a flat or maisonette had 50% higher odds of anxiety and nearly twice the odds of worry about physical health compared with those living in a detached property.

Locality

Living in an urban area rather than a rural or semi-rural location increased the odds of having fatigue, irritability, worry, depression, depressive ideas, somatic symptoms, phobias, worry about physical health, and panic. The odds were around 10% to 40% higher for urban dwellers

for most of these symptoms, but for panic, the odds among urban dwellers were 1.72 times those of rural and semi-rural dwellers.

Notes

1. Sixty three per cent of adults who were in a one-person family unit lived on their own. The other 37% lived in households with at least one other person, although their relationships were such that they were defined as being in separate family units, e.g. flatmates or siblings.

2. On 1st April 1994 the 14 NHS regions were replaced by eight regions. At the time the survey took place however, the 14 regions were still in existence and this is reflected in the relevant tables.

3. See Appendix D for more information on logistic regression and odds ratios.

Table 5.1 Proportion of adults with a score of two or more on each CIS-R symptom by age and sex

	Age										All
	16-19	20-24	25-29	30-34	35-39	40-44	45-49	50-54	55-59	60-64	
	Proportion of adults with a score of 2 or more on each symptom (SE)										
Women											
Fatigue	26 (3)	34 (2)	36 (2)	37 (2)	34 (2)	31 (2)	33 (2)	34 (3)	31 (2)	28 (2)	33 (1)
Sleep problems	23 (3)	30 (2)	25 (2)	25 (2)	26 (2)	28 (2)	28 (2)	38 (2)	31 (2)	33 (2)	28 (1)
Irritability	30 (3)	33 (2)	32 (2)	33 (2)	28 (2)	24 (2)	22 (2)	18 (2)	13 (2)	12 (2)	25 (1)
Worry	22 (3)	27 (2)	3 (2)	25 (2)	24 (2)	26 (2)	22 (2)	22 (2)	19 (2)	14 (2)	23 (1)
Depression	11 (2)	13 (2)	11 (1)	12 (1)	10 (1)	13 (2)	10 (1)	11 (2)	7 (1)	7 (1)	11 (1)
Depressive ideas	14 (2)	14 (2)	12 (1)	12 (1)	11 (1)	12 (2)	11 (1)	12 (2)	6 (1)	5 (1)	11 (1)
Anxiety	10 (2)	9 (1)	9 (1)	11 (1)	11 (1)	11 (1)	12 (1)	16 (2)	11 (1)	11 (1)	11 (1)
Obsessions	10 (2)	14 (2)	13 (1)	12 (1)	12 (1)	12 (2)	10 (1)	13 (2)	10 (1)	6 (1)	12 (1)
Concentration	11 (2)	9 (1)	9 (1)	11 (1)	10 (1)	10 (2)	10 (2)	11 (2)	8 (1)	6 (1)	10 (1)
Somatic symptoms	8 (2)	8 (1)	8 (1)	9 (1)	9 (1)	12 (2)	14 (1)	12 (2)	9 (1)	8 (1)	10 (0)
Compulsions	9 (2)	10 (1)	9 (1)	7 (1)	7 (1)	6 (1)	6 (1)	8 (1)	7 (2)	5 (1)	8 (0)
Phobias	12 (2)	9 (1)	7 (1)	7 (1)	8 (1)	6 (1)	4 (1)	7 (1)	6 (1)	5 (1)	7 (0)
Worry–physical health	4 (1)	5 (1)	5 (1)	6 (1)	5 (1)	4 (1)	4 (1)	6 (1)	4 (1)	5 (1)	5 (0)
Panic	5 (1)	3 (1)	3 (1)	3 (1)	4 (1)	4 (1)	2 (1)	5 (1)	2 (1)	2 (1)	3 (0)
Base	*365*	*555*	*648*	*587*	*531*	*529*	*520*	*413*	*396*	*390*	*4933*
Men											
Fatigue	12 (2)	18 (2)	21 (2)	24 (2)	21 (2)	22 (2)	22 (2)	20 (2)	23 (3)	22 (2)	21 (1)
Sleep problems	22 (3)	19 (2)	20 (2)	20 (2)	23 (2)	21 (2)	19 (2)	20 (2)	24 (2)	23 (2)	21 (1)
Irritability	23 (3)	19 (2)	22 (2)	20 (2)	20 (2)	22 (2)	16 (2)	13 (2)	15 (2)	11 (2)	19 (1)
Worry	11 (2)	19 (2)	17 (2)	19 (2)	21 (2)	18 (2)	16 (2)	17 (2)	15 (2)	13 (2)	17 (1)
Depression	6 (2)	9 (1)	7 (1)	8 (1)	9 (1)	10 (2)	9 (1)	9 (1)	9 (2)	7 (1)	8 (0)
Depressive ideas	7 (2)	8 (1)	6 (1)	7 (1)	7 (1)	7 (1)	7 (1)	6 (1)	7 (1)	8 (1)	7 (0)
Anxiety	5 (1)	7 (1)	9 (1)	8 (1)	10 (1)	9 (2)	7 (1)	9 (2)	10 (2)	6 (1)	8 (0)
Obsessions	7 (2)	7 (1)	6 (1)	6 (1)	8 (1)	9 (1)	7 (1)	6 (1)	5 (1)	6 (1)	7 (0)
Concentration	4 (1)	5 (1)	5 (1)	7 (1)	6 (1)	8 (1)	8 (1)	6 (1)	8 (2)	7 (1)	6 (0)
Somatic symptoms	1 (1)	3 (1)	5 (1)	5 (1)	6 (1)	8 (1)	5 (1)	8 (1)	7 (2)	7 (2)	5 (0)
Compulsions	7 (2)	7 (1)	6 (1)	5 (1)	6 (1)	3 (1)	5 (1)	3 (1)	4 (1)	4 (1)	5 (0)
Phobias	4 (1)	4 (1)	5 (1)	4 (1)	4 (1)	2 (1)	2 (1)	2 (1)	2 (1)	3 (1)	3 (0)
Worry–physical health	1 (1)	2 (1)	3 (1)	3 (1)	6 (1)	6 (1)	5 (1)	6 (1)	8 (2)	6 (1)	4 (0)
Panic	2 (1)	1 (0)	2 (1)	1 (0)	2 (1)	2 (1)	2 (1)	2 (1)	1 (0)	1 (1)	2 (0)
Base	*382*	*569*	*651*	*575*	*505*	*500*	*501*	*415*	*387*	*374*	*4859*
All adults											
Fatigue	19 (2)	26 (2)	28 (1)	30 (1)	28 (2)	27 (2)	28 (2)	27 (2)	27 (2)	25 (2)	27 (1)
Sleep problems	23 (2)	24 (2)	22 (1)	22 (1)	25 (1)	25 (1)	23 (1)	29 (1)	28 (2)	28 (2)	25 (1)
Irritability	27 (2)	26 (2)	27 (1)	26 (1)	24 (1)	23 (1)	19 (1)	15 (1)	14 (1)	12 (1)	22 (1)
Worry	16 (2)	23 (1)	20 (1)	22 (1)	22 (1)	22 (1)	19 (1)	19 (1)	17 (2)	14 (1)	20 (1)
Depression	8 (1)	11 (1)	9 (1)	10 (1)	9 (1)	11 (1)	9 (1)	10 (1)	8 (1)	7 (1)	10 (0)
Depressive ideas	10 (1)	11 (1)	9 (1)	10 (1)	9 (1)	10 (1)	9 (1)	9 (1)	7 (1)	6 (1)	9 (0)
Anxiety	7 (1)	8 (1)	9 (1)	10 (1)	10 (1)	10 (1)	9 (1)	12 (1)	11 (1)	9 (1)	10 (0)
Obsessions	9 (1)	11 (1)	10 (1)	9 (1)	10 (1)	11 (1)	8 (1)	9 (1)	8 (1)	6 (1)	9 (0)
Concentration	8 (1)	7 (1)	7 (1)	9 (1)	8 (1)	9 (1)	9 (1)	8 (1)	8 (1)	6 (1)	8 (0)
Somatic symptoms	4 (1)	6 (1)	6 (1)	7 (1)	8 (1)	10 (1)	9 (1)	10 (1)	8 (1)	8 (1)	8 (0)
Compulsions	8 (1)	8 (1)	7 (1)	6 (1)	6 (1)	4 (1)	6 (1)	5 (1)	6 (1)	4 (1)	6 (0)
Phobias	8 (1)	7 (1)	6 (1)	5 (1)	6 (1)	4 (1)	3 (1)	4 (1)	4 (1)	4 (1)	5 (0)
Worry–physical health	2 (1)	4 (1)	4 (1)	5 (1)	6 (1)	5 (1)	5 (1)	6 (1)	6 (1)	5 (1)	5 (0)
Panic	4 (1)	2 (0)	3 (1)	2 (0)	3 (0)	3 (1)	2 (0)	4 (1)	1 (0)	2 (0)	2 (0)
Base	*747*	*1124*	*1298*	*1161*	*1036*	*1029*	*1021*	*828*	*782*	*765*	*9792*

Table 5.2 Proportion of adults with a score of two or more on each CIS-R symptom by ethnicity and sex

	Ethnicity*			All
	White	West Indian or African	Asian or Oriental	
	Proportion of adults with a score of 2 or more on each symptom (SE)			
Women				
Fatigue	33 (1)	34 (5)	33 (6)	33 (1)
Sleep problems	28 (1)	28 (5)	24 (6)	28 (1)
Irritability	26 (1)	26 (5)	23 (4)	26 (1)
Worry	23 (1)	23 (5)	19 (5)	23 (1)
Depression	10 (1)	21 (4)	18 (4)	11 (1)
Depressive ideas	11 (1)	16 (4)	17 (4)	11 (1)
Anxiety	11 (1)	8 (3)	10 (3)	11 (1)
Obsessions	12 (1)	8 (3)	14 (4)	12 (1)
Concentration and forgetfulness	10 (1)	9 (3)	12 (3)	10 (1)
Somatic symptoms	10 (0)	7 (3)	10 (3)	10 (0)
Compulsions	7 (0)	15 (5)	6 (2)	8 (0)
Phobias	7 (0)	5 (3)	5 (2)	7 (0)
Worry about physical health	4 (0)	6 (3)	13 (3)	5 (0)
Panic	3 (0)	1 (1)	4 (1)	3 (0)
Base	*4633*	*78*	*141*	*4933*
Men				
Fatigue	21 (1)	24 (6)	12 (4)	21 (1)
Sleep problems	21 (1)	20 (5)	16 (3)	21 (1)
Irritability	19 (1)	17 (6)	12 (3)	19 (1)
Worry	17 (1)	23 (6)	17 (3)	17 (1)
Depression	8 (0)	19 (6)	8 (3)	8 (0)
Depressive ideas	7 (0)	16 (6)	10 (3)	7 (0)
Anxiety	8 (0)	8 (4)	7 (2)	8 (0)
Obsessions	7 (0)	13 (4)	8 (4)	7 (0)
Concentration and forgetfulness	6 (0)	12 (5)	7 (2)	6 (0)
Somatic symptoms	5 (0)	5 (3)	3 (2)	5 (0)
Compulsions	5 (0)	7 (3)	2 (1)	5 (0)
Phobias	3 (0)	3 (2)	3 (2)	3 (0)
Worry about physical health	4 (0)	10 (3)	6 (2)	4 (0)
Panic	2 (0)	1 (1)	-	2 (0)
Base	*4546*	*70*	*158*	*4859*
All adults				
Fatigue	27 (1)	29 (4)	22 (4)	27 (1)
Sleep problems	25 (1)	25 (3)	20 (3)	25 (1)
Irritability	22 (1)	22 (4)	17 (3)	22 (1)
Worry	20 (1)	23 (4)	18 (3)	20 (1)
Depression	9 (0)	20 (3)	12 (3)	10 (0)
Depressive ideas	9 (0)	16 (4)	13 (3)	9 (0)
Anxiety	10 (0)	8 (3)	8 (2)	10 (0)
Obsessions	9 (0)	10 (3)	11 (3)	9 (0)
Concentration and forgetfulness	8 (0)	10 (3)	9 (2)	8 (0)
Somatic symptoms	8 (0)	6 (3)	6 (2)	8 (0)
Compulsions	6 (0)	11 (3)	4 (1)	6 (0)
Phobias	5 (0)	4 (2)	4 (1)	5 (0)
Worry about physical health	4 (0)	8 (3)	9 (2)	5 (0)
Panic	3 (0)	1 (1)	2 (1)	2 (0)
Base	*9179*	*148*	*299*	*9792*

*Respondents who could not be classified into the three ethnic groups or refused to answer are included in the "All" category.

Table 5.3 Proportion of adults with a score of two or more on each CIS-R symptom by marital status and sex

	Marital status*						All
	Married	Cohabiting	Single	Widowed	Divorced	Separated	
	Proportion of adults with a score of 2 or more on each symptom (SE)						
Women							
Fatigue	32 (1)	39 (3)	30 (2)	32 (3)	41 (2)	36 (3)	33 (1)
Sleep problems	27 (1)	26 (3)	27 (2)	39 (3)	36 (2)	35 (4)	28 (1)
Irritability	24 (1)	35 (3)	27 (2)	18 (3)	26 (2)	28 (3)	25 (1)
Worry	20 (1)	29 (2)	25 (2)	22 (3)	32 (2)	29 (3)	23 (1)
Depression	9 (1)	14 (2)	12 (1)	15 (2)	13 (1)	16 (2)	11 (1)
Depressive ideas	9 (1)	14 (2)	15 (1)	13 (2)	17 (2)	19 (3)	11 (1)
Anxiety	10 (1)	13 (2)	11 (1)	15 (2)	17 (2)	15 (2)	11 (1)
Obsessions	10 (1)	14 (2)	12 (1)	14 (2)	18 (2)	15 (2)	12 (1)
Concentration	8 (1)	11 (2)	10 (1)	9 (2)	19 (2)	12 (2)	10 (1)
Somatic symptoms	9 (1)	10 (2)	9 (1)	13 (2)	16 (2)	12 (3)	10 (0)
Compulsions	6 (1)	10 (2)	9 (1)	10 (2)	10 (1)	7 (2)	8 (0)
Phobias	5 (0)	10 (2)	10 (1)	5 (1)	11 (2)	8 (2)	7 (0)
Worry– physical health	4 (0)	6 (1)	6 (1)	4 (1)	8 (1)	5 (2)	5 (0)
Panic	3 (0)	3 (1)	4 (1)	6 (2)	5 (1)	5 (1)	3 (0)
Base	*2927*	*362*	*1014*	*171*	*314*	*127*	*4933*
Men							
Fatigue	21 (1)	21 (2)	18 (1)	27 (7)	23 (2)	36 (6)	21 (1)
Sleep problems	20 (1)	18 (2)	22 (1)	37 (6)	26 (3)	36 (5)	21 (1)
Irritability	19 (1)	18 (2)	19 (1)	9 (4)	15 (2)	25 (5)	19 (1)
Worry	16 (1)	20 (2)	16 (1)	16 (5)	21 (3)	34 (6)	17 (1)
Depression	8 (1)	8 (2)	9 (1)	15 (5)	12 (2)	27 (5)	8 (0)
Depressive ideas	6 (0)	6 (1)	8 (1)	10 (4)	10 (2)	21 (4)	7 (0)
Anxiety	8 (0)	8 (1)	8 (1)	6 (3)	10 (2)	21 (5)	8 (0)
Obsessions	6 (1)	8 (1)	8 (1)	6 (3)	11 (2)	16 (4)	7 (0)
Concentration	6 (0)	5 (1)	5 (1)	14 (5)	10 (2)	19 (4)	6 (0)
Somatic symptoms	6 (1)	5 (1)	2 (0)	8 (4)	8 (1)	10 (3)	5 (0)
Compulsions	4 (0)	7 (1)	7 (1)	7 (3)	7 (1)	8 (3)	5 (0)
Phobias	2 (0)	4 (1)	4 (1)	5 (2)	5 (1)	14 (3)	3 (0)
Worry –physical health	5 (0)	5 (1)	2 (0)	13 (4)	6 (1)	7 (3)	4 (0)
Panic	2 (0)	1 (1)	2 (0)	4 (3)	2 (1)	6 (2)	2 (0)
Base	*2868*	*327*	*1343*	*42*	*196*	*56*	*4859*
All adults							
Fatigue	27 (1)	30 (2)	23 (1)	31 (3)	34 (2)	36 (3)	27 (1)
Sleep problems	24 (1)	22 (2)	24 (1)	39 (3)	32 (2)	36 (3)	25 (1)
Irritability	21 (1)	27 (2)	23 (1)	16 (2)	22 (2)	27 (3)	22 (1)
Worry	18 (1)	25 (2)	20 (1)	21 (2)	28 (2)	30 (3)	20 (1)
Depression	8 (0)	11 (1)	10 (1)	15 (2)	12 (1)	20 (2)	10 (0)
Depressive ideas	7 (0)	10 (1)	11 (1)	13 (2)	14 (1)	20 (2)	9 (0)
Anxiety	9 (0)	11 (1)	9 (1)	14 (2)	14 (1)	17 (2)	10 (0)
Obsessions	8 (0)	11 (1)	10 (1)	12 (2)	15 (1)	15 (2)	9 (0)
Concentration	7 (0)	8 (1)	7 (1)	10 (2)	15 (1)	14 (2)	8 (0)
Somatic symptoms	8 (0)	8 (1)	5 (1)	12 (2)	13 (1)	11 (2)	8 (0)
Compulsions	5 (0)	8 (1)	8 (1)	9 (2)	9 (1)	8 (2)	6 (0)
Phobias	4 (0)	8 (1)	7 (1)	5 (1)	9 (1)	10 (2)	5 (0)
Worry –physical health	5 (0)	5 (1)	4 (0)	6 (1)	7 (1)	6 (1)	5 (0)
Panic	2 (0)	2 (1)	3 (0)	5 (1)	4 (1)	5 (1)	2 (0)
Base	*5795*	*688*	*2357*	*213*	*510*	*183*	*9792*

* Respondents with insufficient information to code marital status are included in the "All" category.

Table 5.4 Proportion of adults with a score of two or more on each CIS-R symptom by age when finished full-time education and sex

	Age when finished full-time education*							All
	Not yet finished	14 or under	15	16	17	18	19 or over	
	Proportion of adults with a score of 2 or more on each symptom (SE)							
Women								
Fatigue	27 (4)	34 (2)	36 (2)	32 (1)	31 (2)	32 (2)	33 (2)	33 (1)
Sleep problems	30 (4)	37 (2)	31 (2)	28 (1)	25 (2)	24 (2)	27 (2)	28 (1)
Irritability	32 (4)	18 (2)	24 (1)	27 (1)	26 (2)	26 (2)	25 (2)	25 (1)
Worry	25 (4)	22 (2)	23 (1)	22 (1)	25 (2)	20 (2)	25 (2)	23 (1)
Depression	13 (3)	12 (2)	12 (1)	11 (1)	9 (1)	8 (1)	10 (1)	11 (1)
Depressive ideas	18 (3)	11 (2)	13 (1)	11 (1)	10 (2)	8 (1)	10 (1)	11 (1)
Anxiety	11 (3)	16 (2)	14 (1)	9 (1)	10 (2)	8 (1)	10 (1)	11 (1)
Obsessions	12 (3)	10 (1)	12 (1)	12 (1)	12 (2)	11 (2)	12 (1)	12 (1)
Concentration	14 (3)	10 (2)	11 (1)	10 (1)	9 (1)	7 (1)	8 (1)	10 (1)
Somatic symptoms	7 (2)	11 (1)	12 (1)	9 (1)	6 (1)	9 (1)	11 (1)	10 (0)
Compulsions	13 (3)	7 (1)	9 (1)	7 (1)	8 (1)	6 (1)	5 (1)	8 (0)
Phobias	13 (3)	8 (1)	8 (1)	6 (1)	7 (1)	5 (1)	6 (1)	7 (0)
Worry –physical health	3 (2)	7 (1)	6 (1)	4 (1)	4 (1)	5 (1)	3 (1)	5 (0)
Panic	5 (2)	5 (1)	4 (1)	3 (0)	3 (1)	2 (1)	3 (1)	3 (0)
Base	*241*	*346*	*1135*	*1498*	*496*	*464*	*744*	*4933*
Men								
Fatigue	16 (3)	24 (2)	23 (2)	20 (1)	15 (2)	20 (2)	21 (2)	21 (1)
Sleep problems	30 (3)	24 (2)	24 (2)	18 (1)	19 (2)	18 (2)	20 (2)	21 (1)
Irritability	28 (4)	15 (2)	19 (1)	19 (1)	17 (2)	18 (3)	16 (1)	19 (1)
Worry	14 (3)	15 (2)	18 (1)	16 (1)	14 (2)	16 (2)	19 (2)	17 (1)
Depression	10 (3)	9 (1)	10 (1)	7 (1)	5 (1)	7 (2)	8 (1)	8 (0)
Depressive ideas	11 (3)	9 (2)	8 (1)	7 (1)	4 (1)	5 (1)	6 (1)	7 (0)
Anxiety	9 (2)	10 (2)	10 (1)	7 (1)	7 (1)	9 (2)	8 (1)	8 (0)
Obsessions	8 (3)	8 (2)	7 (1)	7 (1)	7 (1)	6 (1)	6 (1)	7 (0)
Concentration	7 (2)	10 (2)	8 (1)	5 (1)	4 (1)	5 (1)	6 (1)	6 (0)
Somatic symptoms	2 (1)	8 (1)	7 (1)	4 (0)	2 (1)	4 (1)	6 (1)	5 (0)
Compulsions	8 (2)	5 (1)	5 (1)	5 (1)	4 (1)	4 (1)	5 (1)	5 (0)
Phobias	4 (1)	3 (1)	3 (1)	4 (0)	3 (1)	2 (1)	3 (1)	3 (0)
Worry– physical health	2 (1)	8 (1)	6 (1)	3 (0)	3 (1)	5 (1)	4 (1)	4 (0)
Panic	2 (1)	2 (1)	3 (1)	1 (0)	2 (1)	2 (1)	2 (0)	2 (0)
Base	*271*	*354*	*1100*	*1559*	*380*	*339*	*846*	*4859*
All adults								
Fatigue	21 (3)	29 (2)	30 (1)	26 (1)	24 (1)	27 (2)	26 (1)	27 (1)
Sleep problems	30 (3)	30 (2)	27 (1)	23 (1)	22 (2)	22 (2)	23 (1)	25 (1)
Irritability	30 (3)	16 (1)	21 (1)	23 (1)	22 (2)	23 (2)	20 (1)	22 (1)
Worry	19 (2)	18 (1)	20 (1)	19 (1)	20 (1)	18 (1)	22 (1)	20 (1)
Depression	12 (2)	10 (1)	11 (1)	9 (1)	7 (1)	8 (1)	9 (1)	10 (0)
Depressive ideas	14 (2)	10 (1)	10 (1)	9 (1)	8 (1)	7 (1)	8 (1)	9 (0)
Anxiety	10 (2)	13 (1)	12 (1)	8 (0)	9 (1)	8 (1)	9 (1)	10 (0)
Obsessions	10 (2)	9 (1)	9 (1)	9 (1)	10 (1)	9 (1)	9 (1)	9 (0)
Concentration	10 (2)	10 (1)	9 (1)	8 (0)	7 (1)	6 (1)	7 (1)	8 (0)
Somatic symptoms	4 (1)	9 (1)	10 (1)	6 (0)	5 (1)	7 (1)	9 (1)	8 (0)
Compulsions	10 (2)	6 (1)	7 (1)	6 (0)	6 (1)	5 (1)	5 (1)	6 (0)
Phobias	8 (2)	6 (1)	6 (1)	5 (0)	5 (1)	4 (1)	4 (1)	5 (0)
Worry–physical health	3 (1)	8 (1)	6 (1)	4 (0)	4 (1)	5 (1)	4 (0)	5 (0)
Panic	3 (1)	4 (1)	4 (0)	2 (0)	2 (0)	2 (1)	2 (0)	2 (0)
Base	*512*	*700*	*2235*	*3057*	*876*	*804*	*1590*	*9792*

* No answers and those who had never been to school are excluded from the seven age categories but included in the "All" category.

Table 5.5 Proportion of adults with a score of two or more on each CIS-R symptom by educational qualifications and sex

	Educational qualifications						All
	Degree	Teaching, HND, Nursing	A- Level	GCSE, A-C grades or equivalent	GCSE, grades D-F or equivalent	No qualifi- cations	
	Proportion of adults with a score of 2 or more on each symptom (SE)						
Women							
Fatigue	35 (2)	33 (2)	33 (3)	30 (1)	33 (2)	35 (1)	33 (1)
Sleep problems	26 (2)	30 (2)	29 (2)	25 (1)	28 (2)	31 (1)	28 (1)
Irritability	27 (2)	20 (2)	28 (2)	29 (1)	23 (2)	24 (1)	25 (1)
Worry	26 (2)	21 (2)	22 (2)	22 (1)	26 (2)	23 (1)	23 (1)
Depression	10 (1)	7 (1)	10 (1)	9 (1)	10 (1)	13 (1)	11 (1)
Depressive ideas	9 (2)	8 (1)	11 (2)	11 (1)	12 (2)	13 (1)	11 (1)
Anxiety	11 (2)	8 (1)	9 (2)	9 (1)	11 (1)	14 (1)	11 (1)
Obsessions	14 (2)	10 (1)	11 (2)	12 (1)	12 (2)	11 (1)	12 (1)
Concentration	8 (1)	9 (1)	10 (2)	9 (1)	9 (1)	11 (1)	10 (1)
Somatic symptoms	11 (1)	10 (1)	9 (1)	8 (1)	11 (1)	11 (1)	10 (0)
Compulsions	5 (1)	5 (1)	8 (1)	8 (1)	9 (1)	8 (1)	8 (0)
Phobias	5 (1)	5 (1)	6 (1)	7 (1)	9 (1)	7 (1)	7 (0)
Worry –physical health	4 (1)	4 (1)	4 (1)	4 (1)	3 (1)	6 (1)	5 (0)
Panic	3 (1)	2 (1)	2 (1)	3 (0)	4 (1)	4 (1)	3 (0)
Base	*450*	*463*	*442*	*1367*	*587*	*1625*	*4933*
Men							
Fatigue	21 (2)	20 (2)	20 (2)	19 (1)	23 (2)	22 (1)	21 (1)
Sleep problems	18 (2)	19 (2)	21 (2)	23 (1)	18 (2)	23 (1)	21 (1)
Irritability	17 (2)	17 (2)	18 (2)	22 (1)	20 (2)	18 (1)	19 (1)
Worry	20 (2)	15 (1)	17 (2)	15 (1)	17 (2)	18 (1)	17 (1)
Depression	6 (1)	6 (1)	7 (1)	8 (1)	10 (2)	11 (1)	8 (0)
Depressive ideas	6 (1)	4 (1)	7 (1)	7 (1)	6 (1)	9 (1)	7 (0)
Anxiety	10 (1)	5 (1)	10 (1)	7 (1)	9 (1)	9 (1)	8 (0)
Obsessions	7 (1)	6 (1)	7 (1)	7 (1)	6 (1)	7 (1)	7 (0)
Concentration	5 (1)	7 (1)	6 (1)	6 (1)	7 (1)	7 (1)	6 (0)
Somatic symptoms	6 (1)	4 (1)	4 (1)	4 (1)	5 (1)	7 (1)	5 (0)
Compulsions	6 (1)	3 (1)	4 (1)	7 (1)	4 (1)	5 (1)	5 (0)
Phobias	3 (1)	2 (1)	3 (1)	5 (1)	4 (1)	3 (1)	3 (0)
Worry – physical health	2 (1)	4 (1)	3 (1)	4 (1)	3 (1)	8 (1)	4 (0)
Panic	1 (1)	1 (0)	2 (1)	2 (0)	2 (1)	2 (0)	2 (0)
Base	*642*	*695*	*616*	*1174*	*474*	*1258*	*4859*
All adults							
Fatigue	27 (2)	25 (1)	25 (2)	25 (1)	29 (2)	29 (1)	27 (1)
Sleep problems	22 (1)	23 (2)	24 (2)	24 (1)	24 (2)	28 (1)	25 (1)
Irritability	21 (1)	18 (1)	22 (1)	26 (1)	22 (2)	22 (1)	22 (1)
Worry	22 (2)	18 (1)	19 (1)	19 (1)	22 (1)	20 (1)	20 (1)
Depression	8 (1)	7 (1)	8 (1)	9 (1)	10 (1)	12 (1)	10 (0)
Depressive ideas	8 (1)	6 (1)	9 (1)	9 (1)	9 (1)	11 (1)	9 (0)
Anxiety	10 (1)	6 (1)	9 (1)	8 (1)	10 (1)	12 (1)	10 (0)
Obsessions	10 (1)	8 (1)	9 (1)	10 (1)	10 (1)	9 (1)	9 (0)
Concentration	6 (1)	8 (1)	8 (1)	8 (1)	8 (1)	9 (1)	8 (0)
Somatic symptoms	8 (1)	6 (1)	6 (1)	6 (0)	8 (1)	9 (1)	8 (0)
Compulsions	6 (1)	4 (1)	6 (1)	7 (1)	7 (1)	7 (1)	6 (0)
Phobias	4 (1)	3 (1)	4 (1)	6 (1)	7 (1)	5 (0)	5 (0)
Worry–physical health	3 (1)	4 (1)	3 (1)	4 (0)	3 (1)	7 (1)	5 (0)
Panic	2 (0)	1 (0)	2 (1)	2 (0)	3 (0)	4 (0)	2 (0)
Base	*1092*	*1157*	*1058*	*2541*	*1061*	*2883*	*9792*

* For details of educational qualifications see Glossary.

Table 5.6 Proportion of adults with a score of two or more on each CIS-R symptom by employment status and sex

	Employment status				All
	Working full-time	Working part-time	Unemployed	Economically inactive	
	Proportion of adults with a score of 2 or more on each symptom (SE)				
Women					
Fatigue	33 (1)	30 (1)	40 (3)	34 (1)	33 (1)
Sleep problems	24 (1)	27 (1)	39 (3)	32 (1)	28 (1)
Irritability	23 (1)	24 (1)	39 (3)	27 (1)	25 (1)
Worry	22 (1)	20 (1)	38 (3)	23 (1)	23 (1)
Depression	9 (1)	9 (1)	23 (3)	13 (1)	11 (1)
Depressive ideas	8 (1)	10 (1)	25 (3)	13 (1)	11 (1)
Anxiety	9 (1)	8 (1)	20 (3)	14 (1)	11 (1)
Obsessions	10 (1)	10 (1)	26 (3)	12 (1)	12 (1)
Concentration	8 (1)	9 (1)	18 (2)	11 (1)	10 (1)
Somatic symptoms	9 (1)	8 (1)	16 (2)	10 (1)	10 (0)
Compulsions	6 (1)	8 (1)	10 (2)	8 (1)	8 (0)
Phobias	6 (1)	4 (1)	14 (2)	9 (1)	7 (0)
Worry–physical health	3 (0)	3 (0)	7 (1)	7 (1)	5 (0)
Panic	3 (0)	2 (0)	7 (2)	4 (1)	3 (0)
Base	*1713*	*1383*	*268*	*1569*	*4933*
Men					
Fatigue	19 (1)	20 (3)	20 (2)	28 (2)	21 (1)
Sleep problems	17 (1)	27 (3)	28 (2)	33 (2)	21 (1)
Irritability	17 (1)	24 (3)	23 (2)	21 (2)	19 (1)
Worry	15 (1)	16 (3)	24 (2)	20 (2)	17 (1)
Depression	6 (0)	9 (2)	13 (2)	13 (1)	8 (0)
Depressive ideas	5 (0)	8 (2)	14 (2)	12 (1)	7 (0)
Anxiety	6 (0)	10 (2)	13 (1)	13 (1)	8 (0)
Obsessions	6 (0)	8 (2)	10 (1)	10 (2)	7 (0)
Concentration	5 (0)	3 (1)	8 (1)	12 (1)	6 (0)
Somatic symptoms	4 (0)	7 (2)	6 (1)	9 (1)	5 (0)
Compulsions	4 (0)	5 (2)	6 (1)	9 (1)	5 (0)
Phobias	2 (0)	4 (1)	6 (1)	4 (1)	3 (0)
Worry–physical health	3 (0)	2 (1)	7 (1)	9 (1)	4 (0)
Panic	1 (0)	1 (1)	3 (1)	4 (1)	2 (0)
Base	*3290*	*282*	*579*	*708*	*4859*
All adults					
Fatigue	24 (1)	28 (1)	26 (2)	32 (1)	27 (1)
Sleep problems	19 (1)	27 (1)	31 (2)	32 (1)	25 (1)
Irritability	19 (1)	24 (1)	28 (2)	25 (1)	22 (1)
Worry	18 (1)	20 (1)	28 (2)	22 (1)	20 (1)
Depression	7 (0)	9 (1)	16 (2)	13 (1)	10 (0)
Depressive ideas	6 (0)	10 (1)	17 (1)	13 (1)	9 (0)
Anxiety	7 (0)	8 (1)	15 (1)	14 (1)	10 (0)
Obsessions	7 (0)	10 (1)	15 (1)	12 (1)	9 (0)
Concentration	6 (0)	8 (1)	11 (1)	11 (1)	8 (0)
Somatic symptoms	6 (0)	8 (1)	9 (1)	10 (1)	8 (0)
Compulsions	5 (0)	7 (1)	7 (1)	8 (1)	6 (0)
Phobias	4 (0)	4 (1)	9 (1)	8 (1)	5 (0)
Worry–physical health	3 (0)	3 (0)	7 (1)	8 (1)	5 (0)
Panic	2 (0)	2 (0)	4 (1)	4 (0)	2 (0)
Base	*5003*	*1666*	*847*	*2276*	*9792*

Table 5.7 Proportion of adults with a score of two or more on each CIS-R symptom by social class (based on occupation of head of family unit) and sex

	Social class*						All§
	I	II	IIINM	IIIM	IV	V	
	Proportion of adults with a score of 2 or more on each symptom (SE)						
Women							
Fatigue	35 (3)	31 (1)	31 (2)	35 (2)	34 (2)	33 (3)	33 (1)
Sleep problems	27 (3)	27 (2)	28 (2)	28 (1)	31 (2)	30 (3)	28 (1)
Irritability	25 (2)	22 (1)	25 (2)	27 (1)	26 (2)	34 (3)	25 (1)
Worry	23 (2)	22 (1)	24 (2)	22 (1)	25 (2)	25 (3)	23 (1)
Depression	9 (2)	7 (1)	11 (1)	11 (1)	13 (1)	16 (3)	11 (1)
Depressive ideas	8 (1)	8 (1)	12 (1)	11 (1)	15 (2)	17 (3)	11 (1)
Anxiety	10 (2)	9 (1)	11 (1)	11 (1)	12 (1)	16 (3)	11 (1)
Obsessions	15 (2)	10 (1)	12 (1)	11 (1)	10 (1)	14 (2)	12 (1)
Concentration	9 (2)	9 (1)	9 (1)	9 (1)	11 (1)	14 (2)	10 (1)
Somatic symptoms	9 (2)	9 (1)	12 (1)	9 (1)	9 (1)	13 (2)	10 (0)
Compulsions	5 (1)	6 (1)	8 (1)	8 (1)	10 (1)	7 (1)	8 (0)
Phobias	4 (1)	5 (1)	8 (1)	6 (1)	9 (1)	10 (2)	7 (0)
Worry–physical health	3 (1)	3 (1)	6 (1)	5 (1)	5 (1)	7 (2)	5 (0)
Panic	1 (1)	2 (0)	4 (1)	4 (1)	4 (1)	6 (2)	3 (0)
Base	*285*	*1332*	*869*	*1263*	*782*	*245*	*4933*
Men							
Fatigue	19 (2)	22 (1)	20 (2)	21 (1)	21 (2)	19 (3)	21 (1)
Sleep problems	14 (2)	20 (1)	22 (2)	21 (1)	22 (2)	25 (3)	21 (1)
Irritability	16 (2)	17 (1)	20 (2)	19 (1)	20 (2)	20 (3)	18 (1)
Worry	16 (2)	18 (1)	19 (2)	16 (1)	16 (2)	20 (3)	17 (1)
Depression	6 (1)	7 (1)	11 (2)	8 (1)	9 (1)	10 (2)	8 (0)
Depressive ideas	3 (1)	6 (1)	9 (1)	7 (1)	7 (1)	8 (2)	7 (0)
Anxiety	5 (1)	8 (1)	11 (1)	8 (1)	8 (1)	9 (2)	8 (0)
Obsessions	5 (1)	8 (1)	6 (1)	7 (1)	6 (1)	7 (2)	7 (0)
Concentration	4 (1)	8 (1)	7 (1)	6 (1)	5 (1)	7 (2)	6 (0)
Somatic symptoms	4 (1)	6 (1)	4 (1)	5 (1)	6 (1)	6 (2)	5 (0)
Compulsions	3 (1)	5 (1)	5 (1)	5 (1)	6 (1)	3 (1)	5 (0)
Phobias	2 (1)	3 (0)	4 (1)	3 (0)	4 (1)	4 (1)	3 (0)
Worry–physical health	2 (1)	5 (1)	4 (1)	5 (1)	5 (1)	6 (2)	4 (0)
Panic	-	2 (0)	1 (0)	2 (0)	2 (1)	3 (1)	2 (0)
Base	*364*	*1222*	*614*	*1514*	*700*	*266*	*4859*
All adults							
Fatigue	26 (2)	26 (1)	27 (1)	27 (1)	28 (1)	26 (2)	27 (1)
Sleep problems	20 (2)	24 (1)	26 (1)	24 (1)	26 (1)	28 (2)	25 (1)
Irritability	20 (2)	19 (1)	23 (1)	22 (1)	23 (1)	27 (2)	22 (1)
Worry	19 (2)	20 (1)	22 (1)	18 (1)	20 (1)	22 (2)	20 (1)
Depression	7 (1)	7 (1)	11 (1)	10 (1)	11 (1)	13 (2)	9 (0)
Depressive ideas	5 (1)	7 (1)	11 (1)	9 (1)	11 (1)	12 (1)	9 (0)
Anxiety	7 (1)	9 (1)	11 (1)	9 (1)	10 (1)	13 (2)	10 (0)
Obsessions	10 (1)	9 (1)	10 (1)	9 (1)	8 (1)	10 (2)	9 (0)
Concentration	6 (1)	8 (1)	8 (1)	7 (1)	8 (1)	10 (1)	8 (0)
Somatic symptoms	6 (1)	8 (1)	9 (1)	7 (0)	7 (1)	9 (1)	8 (0)
Compulsions	4 (1)	5 (0)	7 (1)	6 (0)	8 (1)	5 (1)	6 (0)
Phobias	3 (1)	4 (0)	6 (1)	5 (0)	7 (1)	7 (1)	5 (0)
Worry physical health	2 (1)	4 (0)	5 (1)	5 (0)	5 (1)	6 (1)	5 (0)
Panic	0 (0)	2 (0)	3 (0)	3 (0)	3 (0)	4 (1)	2 (0)
Base	*649*	*2554*	*1484*	*2776*	*1482*	*511*	*9792*

* I = Professional; II = Employers and Managers; IIINM = Intermediate and junior non manual IIIM – Skilled manual and own account non-professional; IV = semi skilled manual and personal service; V = Unskilled manual.

§ No answers, members of the Armed Forces, full-time students and those who have never worked are excluded from the six social class categories but included in the "All" category.

Table 5.8   Proportion of adults with a score of two or more on each CIS-R symptom by family unit type and sex

	Family unit type*						All
	Couple, no child	Couple & child(ren)	Lone parent & child(ren)	One person only	Adult with parents	Adult with one parent	

Proportion of adults with a score of 2 or more on each symptom (SE)

Women							
Fatigue	31 (1)	34 (1)	40 (2)	36 (2)	21 (3)	26 (5)	33 (1)
Sleep problems	30 (1)	26 (1)	35 (2)	34 (2)	22 (3)	25 (5)	28 (1)
Irritability	19 (1)	29 (1)	32 (2)	21 (2)	27 (3)	21 (5)	25 (1)
Worry	20 (1)	22 (1)	28 (2)	29 (2)	22 (3)	24 (4)	23 (1)
Depression	8 (1)	11 (1)	15 (1)	14 (1)	10 (2)	10 (3)	11 (1)
Depressive ideas	7 (1)	10 (1)	20 (1)	15 (1)	11 (2)	14 (4)	11 (1)
Anxiety	10 (1)	10 (1)	15 (1)	14 (1)	8 (2)	9 (3)	11 (1)
Obsessions	11 (1)	10 (1)	16 (2)	16 (1)	7 (2)	13 (3)	12 (1)
Concentration	7 (1)	10 (1)	13 (1)	14 (1)	6 (2)	13 (4)	10 (1)
Somatic symptoms	8 (1)	10 (1)	14 (2)	13 (1)	7 (2)	4 (2)	10 (0)
Compulsions	7 (1)	6 (1)	11 (1)	9 (1)	8 (2)	8 (3)	8 (0)
Phobias	5 (1)	6 (1)	10 (1)	10 (1)	9 (2)	9 (3)	7 (0)
Worry –physical health	5 (1)	4 (0)	6 (1)	8 (1)	2 (1)	6 (3)	5 (0)
Panic	3 (0)	3 (0)	5 (1)	4 (1)	5 (1)	1 (1)	3 (0)
Base	*1342*	*1957*	*502*	*593*	*424*	*115*	*4933*
Men							
Fatigue	21 (1)	22 (1)	28 (6)	25 (2)	15 (2)	13 (3)	21 (1)
Sleep problems	20 (1)	20 (1)	24 (5)	27 (2)	21 (2)	17 (3)	21 (1)
Irritability	15 (1)	21 (1)	19 (5)	16 (1)	22 (2)	21 (3)	19 (1)
Worry	16 (1)	17 (1)	26 (5)	20 (1)	14 (2)	16 (3)	17 (1)
Depression	7 (1)	8 (1)	12 (4)	10 (1)	8 (2)	12 (3)	8 (0)
Depressive ideas	5 (1)	6 (1)	13 (4)	10 (1)	7 (1)	9 (2)	7 (0)
Anxiety	7 (1)	8 (1)	13 (4)	12 (1)	5 (1)	8 (2)	8 (0)
Obsessions	6 (1)	6 (1)	8 (3)	11 (1)	6 (1)	7 (2)	7 (0)
Concentration	6 (1)	7 (1)	9 (3)	9 (1)	4 (1)	5 (2)	6 (0)
Somatic symptoms	6 (1)	6 (1)	5 (2)	6 (1)	1 (1)	2 (1)	5 (0)
Compulsions	5 (1)	4 (0)	10 (3)	7 (1)	5 (1)	10 (2)	5 (0)
Phobias	3 (0)	2 (0)	5 (2)	6 (1)	4 (1)	6 (2)	3 (0)
Worry–physical health	5 (1)	5 (1)	5 (2)	5 (1)	1 (1)	3 (1)	4 (0)
Panic	2 (0)	1 (0)	5 (2)	2 (0)	1 (1)	4 (2)	2 (0)
Base	*1237*	*1974*	*63*	*724*	*664*	*198*	*4859*
All adults							
Fatigue	26 (1)	28 (1)	39 (2)	30 (1)	17 (2)	18 (3)	27 (1)
Sleep problems	25 (1)	22 (1)	34 (2)	30 (1)	21 (2)	20 (3)	25 (1)
Irritability	17 (1)	25 (1)	30 (2)	18 (1)	24 (2)	21 (3)	22 (1)
Worry	18 (1)	19 (1)	27 (1)	24 (1)	17 (2)	19 (3)	20 (1)
Depression	7 (1)	9 (1)	14 (1)	12 (1)	9 (1)	11 (2)	10 (0)
Depressive ideas	6 (0)	8 (1)	19 (1)	12 (1)	9 (1)	11 (2)	9 (0)
Anxiety	8 (1)	9 (1)	15 (1)	13 (1)	6 (1)	9 (2)	10 (0)
Obsessions	9 (1)	8 (0)	15 (1)	13 (1)	6 (1)	9 (2)	9 (0)
Concentration	6 (0)	8 (0)	13 (1)	12 (1)	5 (1)	8 (2)	8 (0)
Somatic symptoms	7 (1)	8 (0)	13 (1)	9 (1)	4 (1)	3 (1)	8 (0)
Compulsions	6 (0)	5 (0)	11 (1)	8 (1)	6 (1)	10 (2)	6 (0)
Phobias	4 (0)	4 (0)	9 (1)	8 (1)	6 (1)	7 (2)	5 (0)
Worry–physical health	5 (0)	4 (0)	6 (1)	6 (1)	2 (1)	4 (1)	5 (0)
Panic	2 (0)	2 (0)	5 (1)	3 (0)	3 (1)	3 (1)	2 (0)
Base	*2578*	*3931*	*564*	*1317*	*1088*	*313*	*9792*

* For details of family unit type, see Glossary.

Table 5.9 Proportion of adults with a score of two or more on each CIS-R symptom by tenure and sex

	Tenure				All
	Owned	Owned with mortgage	Rented from LA or HA	Rented from other source	
	Proportion of adults with a score of 2 or more on each symptom (SE)				
Women					
Fatigue	28 (2)	31 (1)	41 (2)	36 (3)	33 (1)
Sleep problems	29 (2)	26 (1)	32 (2)	32 (2)	28 (1)
Irritability	18 (1)	26 (1)	31 (2)	28 (3)	25 (1)
Worry	18 (1)	22 (1)	28 (2)	27 (2)	23 (1)
Depression	7 (1)	9 (1)	16 (1)	13 (2)	11 (1)
Depressive ideas	6 (1)	10 (1)	17 (1)	15 (2)	11 (1)
Anxiety	8 (1)	9 (1)	17 (1)	13 (2)	11 (1)
Obsessions	8 (1)	12 (1)	14 (1)	15 (2)	12 (1)
Concentration and forgetfulness	8 (1)	9 (1)	12 (1)	12 (2)	10 (1)
Somatic symptoms	7 (1)	10 (1)	11 (1)	9 (1)	10 (0)
Compulsions	6 (1)	7 (1)	10 (1)	8 (1)	8 (0)
Phobias	6 (1)	6 (0)	11 (1)	8 (1)	7 (0)
Worry about physical health	4 (1)	4 (0)	8 (1)	3 (1)	5 (0)
Panic	3 (1)	3 (0)	6 (1)	3 (1)	3 (0)
Base	842	2659	1008	424	4933
Men					
Fatigue	18 (2)	19 (1)	26 (2)	25 (2)	21 (1)
Sleep problems	18 (2)	19 (1)	25 (2)	25 (2)	21 (1)
Irritability	13 (1)	19 (1)	23 (1)	20 (2)	19 (1)
Worry	11 (1)	16 (1)	22 (2)	20 (2)	17 (1)
Depression	8 (1)	7 (1)	14 (1)	8 (1)	8 (0)
Depressive ideas	4 (1)	6 (1)	13 (1)	8 (1)	7 (0)
Anxiety	7 (1)	7 (1)	13 (1)	11 (2)	8 (0)
Obsessions	5 (1)	6 (1)	8 (1)	10 (1)	7 (0)
Concentration and forgetfulness	4 (1)	6 (1)	10 (1)	7 (1)	6 (0)
Somatic symptoms	4 (1)	5 (0)	8 (1)	6 (1)	5 (0)
Compulsions	4 (1)	4 (0)	8 (1)	6 (1)	5 (0)
Phobias	2 (1)	2 (0)	6 (1)	4 (1)	3 (0)
Worry about physical health	4 (1)	4 (0)	7 (1)	5 (1)	4 (0)
Panic	2 (0)	1 (0)	4 (1)	2 (1)	2 (0)
Base	752	2834	792	481	4859
All adults					
Fatigue	23 (1)	25 (1)	34 (1)	30 (2)	27 (1)
Sleep problems	24 (1)	23 (1)	29 (1)	28 (2)	25 (1)
Irritability	15 (1)	22 (1)	27 (1)	24 (2)	22 (1)
Worry	14 (1)	19 (1)	26 (1)	23 (1)	20 (1)
Depression	7 (1)	8 (0)	15 (1)	10 (1)	10 (0)
Depressive ideas	5 (1)	8 (0)	15 (1)	12 (1)	9 (0)
Anxiety	7 (1)	8 (0)	15 (1)	12 (1)	10 (0)
Obsessions	7 (1)	8 (0)	11 (1)	12 (1)	9 (0)
Concentration and forgetfulness	6 (1)	7 (0)	11 (1)	10 (1)	8 (0)
Somatic symptoms	6 (1)	7 (0)	9 (1)	7 (1)	8 (0)
Compulsions	5 (0)	6 (0)	9 (1)	7 (1)	6 (0)
Phobias	4 (1)	4 (0)	9 (1)	6 (1)	5 (0)
Worry about physical health	4 (0)	4 (0)	8 (1)	4 (1)	5 (0)
Panic	2 (0)	2 (0)	5 (1)	3 (1)	2 (0)
Base	1595	5493	1800	905	9792

49

Table 5.10 Proportion of adults with a score of two or more on each CIS-R symptom by type of accommodation and sex

	Type of accommodation				All
	Detached	Semi-detached	Terraced	Flat or maisonette	
	Proportion of adults with a score of 2 or more on each symptom (SE)				
Women					
Fatigue	30 (1)	30 (1)	35 (1)	39 (2)	33 (1)
Sleep problems	28 (2)	26 (1)	29 (1)	32 (2)	28 (1)
Irritability	20 (1)	24 (1)	30 (1)	27 (2)	25 (1)
Worry	20 (1)	20 (1)	25 (1)	29 (2)	23 (1)
Depression	7 (1)	10 (1)	12 (1)	14 (1)	11 (1)
Depressive ideas	7 (1)	11 (1)	12 (1)	16 (1)	11 (1)
Anxiety	9 (1)	9 (1)	11 (1)	17 (1)	11 (1)
Obsessions	11 (1)	11 (1)	12 (1)	14 (1)	12 (1)
Concentration and forgetfulness	8 (1)	8 (1)	12 (1)	10 (1)	10 (1)
Somatic symptoms	8 (1)	10 (1)	10 (1)	11 (1)	10 (0)
Compulsions	5 (1)	7 (1)	9 (1)	9 (1)	8 (0)
Phobias	5 (1)	6 (1)	8 (1)	9 (1)	7 (0)
Worry about physical health	3 (1)	4 (0)	6 (1)	7 (1)	5 (0)
Panic	2 (1)	3 (0)	4 (0)	4 (1)	3 (0)
Base	*1075*	*1582*	*1518*	*758*	*4933*
Men					
Fatigue	19 (1)	20 (1)	22 (1)	24 (2)	21 (1)
Sleep problems	18 (1)	21 (1)	20 (1)	26 (2)	21 (1)
Irritability	17 (2)	17 (1)	21 (1)	20 (1)	19 (1)
Worry	17 (1)	15 (1)	17 (1)	21 (1)	17 (1)
Depression	8 (1)	8 (1)	9 (1)	11 (1)	8 (0)
Depressive ideas	6 (1)	7 (1)	7 (1)	10 (1)	7 (0)
Anxiety	5 (1)	8 (1)	9 (1)	12 (1)	8 (0)
Obsessions	6 (1)	6 (1)	7 (1)	10 (1)	7 (0)
Concentration and forgetfulness	5 (1)	6 (1)	6 (1)	10 (1)	6 (0)
Somatic symptoms	5 (1)	4 (1)	6 (1)	7 (1)	5 (0)
Compulsions	4 (1)	4 (1)	6 (1)	6 (1)	5 (0)
Phobias	2 (1)	3 (1)	4 (1)	6 (1)	3 (0)
Worry about physical health	3 (1)	4 (1)	5 (1)	8 (1)	4 (0)
Panic	1 (0)	1 (0)	2 (0)	3 (1)	2 (0)
Base	*1038*	*1679*	*1441*	*701*	*4859*
All adults					
Fatigue	24 (1)	25 (1)	28 (1)	31 (1)	27 (1)
Sleep problems	23 (1)	24 (1)	25 (1)	29 (1)	25 (1)
Irritability	19 (1)	20 (1)	26 (1)	23 (1)	22 (1)
Worry	19 (1)	17 (1)	21 (1)	25 (1)	20 (1)
Depression	8 (1)	9 (1)	10 (1)	13 (1)	10 (0)
Depressive ideas	7 (1)	9 (1)	10 (1)	13 (1)	9 (0)
Anxiety	7 (1)	8 (1)	10 (1)	14 (1)	10 (0)
Obsessions	8 (1)	8 (1)	10 (1)	12 (1)	9 (0)
Concentration and forgetfulness	7 (1)	7 (1)	9 (1)	10 (1)	8 (0)
Somatic symptoms	6 (1)	7 (0)	8 (0)	9 (1)	8 (0)
Compulsions	5 (1)	6 (1)	7 (1)	8 (1)	6 (0)
Phobias	4 (1)	4 (0)	6 (0)	7 (1)	5 (0)
Worry about physical health	3 (0)	4 (0)	5 (0)	8 (1)	5 (0)
Panic	2 (0)	2 (0)	3 (0)	4 (0)	2 (0)
Base	*2113*	*3261*	*1960*	*1458*	*9792*

Table 5.11 Proportion of adults with a score of two or more on each CIS-R symptom by Regional Health Authority (RHA) and sex

	RHA								
	Northern	Yorkshire	Trent	East Anglia	NW Thames	NE Thames	SE Thames	SW Thames	Wessex
	Proportion of adults with a score of two or more on each symptom (SE)								
Women									
Fatigue	34 (1)	36 (3)	29 (2)	28 (5)	33 (4)	40 (3)	36 (3)	37 (4)	26 (4)
Sleep problems	34 (2)	30 (3)	26 (3)	27 (2)	24 (2)	28 (2)	32 (3)	32 (3)	21 (3)
Irritability	27 (3)	29 (3)	22 (2)	22 (2)	22 (2)	29 (2)	29 (3)	26 (3)	23 (3)
Worry	23 (3)	24 (4)	17 (2)	22 (2)	22 (3)	29 (3)	30 (3)	25 (4)	19 (3)
Depression	8 (1)	12 (3)	7 (2)	9 (2)	13 (2)	15 (3)	11 (2)	8 (1)	10 (1)
Depressive ideas	12 (2)	12 (3)	7 (1)	11 (2)	12 (3)	18 (3)	11 (2)	12 (2)	8 (2)
Anxiety	11 (2)	13 (2)	8 (1)	13 (4)	10 (2)	15 (2)	11 (2)	9 (3)	9 (2)
Obsessions	13 (2)	12 (3)	8 (2)	11 (2)	13 (2)	12 (1)	14 (2)	13 (3)	14 (3)
Concentration	10 (2)	11 (2)	7 (1)	10 (3)	9 (1)	11 (3)	12 (2)	10 (3)	6 (2)
Somatic symptoms	8 (1)	12 (2)	7 (1)	9 (3)	12 (2)	17 (2)	12 (1)	9 (2)	9 (1)
Compulsions	6 (2)	8 (1)	6 (1)	7 (3)	8 (3)	9 (2)	6 (2)	8 (2)	8 (2)
Phobias	7 (2)	7 (1)	5 (1)	6 (2)	6 (1)	8 (2)	10 (1)	12 (2)	8 (2)
Worry–physical health	6 (2)	7 (1)	4 (1)	2 (1)	6 (2)	6 (1)	5 (1)	4 (2)	4 (1)
Panic	5 (1)	4 (1)	2 (1)	2 (1)	3 (1)	5 (1)	2 (1)	3 (1)	3 (1)
Base	*262*	*352*	*429*	*207*	*318*	*308*	*354*	*255*	*299*
Men									
Fatigue	23 (3)	20 (2)	21 (2)	18 (2)	20 (3)	19 (2)	20 (2)	21 (3)	20 (3)
Sleep problems	23 (3)	20 (3)	22 (3)	15 (4)	21 (3)	20 (2)	20 (3)	25 (3)	21 (3)
Irritability	17 (3)	19 (2)	18 (2)	15 (4)	18 (2)	25 (3)	22 (3)	22 (2)	16 (3)
Worry	15 (1)	14 (2)	17 (2)	10 (3)	18 (3)	21 (2)	17 (2)	23 (2)	17 (2)
Depression	9 (2)	6 (1)	9 (1)	4 (2)	8 (1)	10 (2)	11 (2)	8 (2)	8 (2)
Depressive ideas	8 (2)	8 (1)	7 (1)	2 (1)	7 (1)	9 (2)	6 (1)	8 (2)	8 (2)
Anxiety	8 (2)	8 (1)	7 (1)	5 (2)	7 (1)	12 (2)	8 (2)	13 (3)	5 (1)
Obsessions	8 (2)	4 (1)	6 (2)	6 (2)	10 (1)	6 (2)	8 (2)	6 (2)	8 (1)
Concentration	4 (1)	8 (2)	6 (1)	2 (1)	9 (1)	7 (2)	6 (2)	6 (1)	6 (1)
Somatic symptoms	5 (2)	3 (1)	6 (1)	1 (1)	7 (2)	5 (1)	5 (1)	4 (1)	5 (2)
Compulsions	6 (2)	3 (1)	6 (1)	3 (1)	6 (1)	5 (1)	5 (1)	5 (1)	4 (1)
Phobias	1 (0)	2 (1)	3 (1)	2 (1)	4 (1)	3 (1)	2 (1)	4 (1)	5 (2)
Worry–physical health	5 (1)	6 (1)	4 (1)	4 (2)	4 (1)	5 (1)	5 (1)	4 (1)	3 (1)
Panic	1 (1)	2 (1)	2 (1)	1 (1)	2 (1)	2 (1)	2 (1)	1 (1)	1 (1)
Base	*265*	*331*	*498*	*173*	*327*	*325*	*327*	*269*	*294*
All adults									
Fatigue	28 (2)	8 (2)	24 (2)	23 (3)	26 (2)	29 (2)	28 (2)	29 (2)	23 (3)
Sleep problems	29 (1)	5 (2)	24 (2)	22 (3)	22 (1)	24 (2)	26 (2)	28 (2)	21 (3)
Irritability	22 (2)	4 (2)	20 (2)	19 (3)	20 (2)	27 (2)	25 (2)	24 (2)	20 (2)
Worry	19 (2)	9 (2)	17 (1)	17 (2)	20 (2)	25 (2)	24 (2)	24 (3)	18 (2)
Depression	8 (2)	9 (2)	8 (1)	7 (2)	11 (2)	13 (1)	11 (1)	8 (1)	9 (1)
Depressive ideas	10 (2)	0 (2)	7 (1)	7 (1)	10 (2)	13 (2)	9 (1)	10 (1)	8 (1)
Anxiety	10 (1)	1 (1)	8 (1)	9 (3)	9 (1)	14 (2)	10 (1)	11 (2)	7 (2)
Obsessions	10 (2)	8 (2)	7 (2)	9 (2)	11 (2)	9 (1)	11 (2)	9 (2)	11 (2)
Concentration	7 (1)	0 (1)	7 (1)	7 (2)	9 (1)	9 (1)	9 (1)	8 (2)	6 (1)
Somatic symptoms	7 (1)	8 (1)	6 (1)	6 (1)	9 (1)	11 (1)	9 (1)	7 (1)	7 (1)
Compulsions	6 (1)	6 (1)	6 (1)	5 (2)	7 (1)	7 (1)	6 (1)	6 (1)	6 (1)
Phobias	4 (1)	5 (1)	4 (1)	4 (1)	5 (1)	5 (1)	6 (1)	8 (1)	6 (1)
Worry–physical health	6 (1)	6 (1)	4 (1)	3 (1)	5 (1)	5 (1)	5 (1)	4 (1)	3 (1)
Panic	3 (1)	3 (1)	2 (0)	1 (1)	2 (1)	3 (1)	2 (0)	2 (1)	2 (0)
Base	*527*	*683*	*927*	*380*	*644*	*634*	*680*	*524*	*594*

Oxford	South Western	West Midlands	Mersey	North Western	England	Scotland	Wales	All	
									Women
26 (4)	33 (4)	33 (3)	38 (5)	32 (4)	33 (1)	31 (3)	38 (4)	33 (1)	Fatigue
30 (5)	27 (2)	30 (3)	31 (5)	28 (2)	28 (1)	26 (4)	31 (3)	28 (1)	Sleep problems
22 (4)	21 (2)	28 (3)	30 (3)	26 (3)	26 (1)	24 (2)	26 (2)	25 (1)	Irritability
18 (3)	21 (2)	26 (3)	27 (3)	18 (2)	23 (1)	22 (2)	23 (2)	23 (1)	Worry
7 (2)	8 (1)	13 (2)	11 (2)	13 (2)	10 (1)	12 (2)	13 (2)	11 (1)	Depression
5 (2)	9 (2)	12 (2)	13 (2)	13 (2)	11 (1)	10 (2)	14 (4)	11 (1)	Depressive ideas
7 (1)	9 (1)	11 (1)	13 (2)	11 (2)	11 (1)	10 (2)	14 (4)	11 (1)	Anxiety
10 (2)	8 (2)	14 (2)	14 (2)	8 (1)	12 (1)	9 (2)	14 (1)	12 (1)	Obsessions
9 (2)	6 (2)	12 (2)	9 (1)	11 (2)	10 (1)	9 (2)	11 (3)	10 (1)	Concentration
4 (1)	11 (2)	10 (1)	9 (1)	9 (1)	10 (0)	7 (1)	8 (2)	10 (0)	Somatic symptoms
7 (1)	3 (1)	9 (2)	9 (3)	7 (2)	8 (1)	6 (1)	10 (2)	8 (0)	Compulsions
7 (1)	6 (1)	7 (1)	7 (2)	6 (1)	7 (0)	6 (2)	7 (2)	7 (0)	Phobias
3 (1)	4 (1)	5 (1)	9 (2)	4 (1)	5 (0)	4 (1)	6 (1)	5 (0)	Worry–physical health
3 (1)	2 (1)	4 (1)	5 (2)	5 (1)	3 (0)	4 (1)	3 (2)	3 (0)	Panic
243	*259*	*434*	*234*	*362*	*4317*	*362*	*254*	*4933*	*Base*
									Men
18 (5)	17 (3)	23 (2)	27 (3)	21 (3)	21 (1)	20 (3)	23 (3)	21 (1)	Fatigue
18 (4)	20 (3)	22 (2)	18 (3)	23 (3)	21 (1)	22 (2)	20 (3)	21 (1)	Sleep problems
13 (3)	16 (3)	19 (2)	25 (3)	20 (3)	19 (1)	16 (2)	19 (3)	19 (1)	Irritability
16 (4)	16 (2)	16 (2)	20 (3)	18 (2)	17 (1)	15 (2)	14 (3)	17 (1)	Worry
7 (2)	6 (2)	10 (1)	7 (1)	11 (2)	8 (0)	7 (1)	10 (1)	8 (0)	Depression
6 (2)	5 (1)	9 (2)	6 (2)	6 (1)	7 (0)	5 (1)	7 (1)	7 (0)	Depressive ideas
8 (3)	5 (1)	10 (1)	10 (2)	8 (1)	8 (0)	8 (2)	8 (2)	8 (0)	Anxiety
8 (1)	9 (2)	9 (2)	6 (2)	3 (1)	7 (0)	7 (1)	7 (3)	7 (0)	Obsessions
6 (2)	5 (1)	7 (1)	6 (2)	8 (1)	6 (0)	5 (2)	7 (1)	6 (0)	Concentration
5 (2)	6 (2)	7 (1)	5 (2)	6 (1)	5 (0)	7 (2)	5 (1)	5 (0)	Somatic symptoms
4 (2)	5 (1)	6 (1)	4 (1)	5 (1)	5 (0)	6 (2)	6 (3)	5 (0)	Compulsions
4 (2)	4 (1)	3 (1)	6 (2)	3 (1)	3 (0)	3 (1)	4 (2)	3 (0)	Phobias
4 (2)	4 (1)	4 (1)	4 (2)	4 (1)	4 (0)	7 (2)	5 (1)	4 (0)	Worry–physical health
1 (1)	1 (0)	2 (1)	3 (1)	3 (1)	2 (0)	1 (0)	0 (0)	2 (0)	Panic
259	*261*	*429*	*200*	*339*	*4297*	*316*	*245*	*4859*	*Base*
									All Adults
22 (4)	25 (2)	28 (2)	33 (2)	27 (3)	27 (1)	26 (2)	30 (3)	27 (1)	Fatigue
24 (4)	23 (2)	26 (2)	25 (4)	26 (2)	25 (1)	24 (3)	26 (2)	25 (1)	Sleep problems
17 (3)	19 (2)	23 (2)	28 (3)	23 (2)	22 (1)	21 (2)	22 (2)	22 (1)	Irritability
17 (3)	18 (2)	21 (2)	24 (3)	18 (1)	20 (1)	19 (1)	19 (2)	20 (0)	Worry
7 (2)	7 (1)	11 (1)	9 (1)	12 (2)	9 (0)	10 (1)	12 (1)	10 (0)	Depression
6 (2)	7 (1)	11 (1)	10 (2)	10 (1)	9 (0)	8 (1)	10 (2)	9 (0)	Depressive ideas
8 (2)	7 (1)	10 (1)	12 (2)	10 (1)	10 (0)	9 (1)	11 (2)	10 (0)	Anxiety
9 (1)	9 (1)	11 (1)	10 (1)	6 (1)	9 (0)	8 (1)	10 (2)	9 (0)	Obsessions
8 (2)	6 (1)	10 (1)	8 (1)	9 (1)	8 (0)	7 (2)	9 (2)	8 (0)	Concentration
4 (1)	8 (1)	8 (1)	7 (1)	7 (1)	8 (0)	7 (1)	6 (1)	8 (0)	Somatic symptoms
5 (1)	4 (1)	8 (1)	7 (2)	6 (1)	6 (0)	6 (1)	8 (2)	6 (0)	Compulsions
6 (1)	5 (1)	5 (1)	7 (1)	5 (0)	5 (0)	4 (1)	6 (1)	5 (0)	Phobias
4 (2)	4 (1)	4 (1)	7 (2)	4 (1)	4 (0)	5 (1)	6 (1)	5 (0)	Worry–physical health
2 (1)	1 (0)	3 (1)	4 (1)	4 (1)	2 (0)	3 (1)	2 (1)	2 (0)	Panic
502	*520*	*863*	*434*	*701*	*8614*	*678*	*499*	*9792*	*Base*

Table 5.12   Proportion of adults with a score of two or more on each CIS-R symptom by locality and sex

	Locality			All
	Urban	Semi-rural	Rural	
	Proportion of adults with a score of 2 or more on each symptom (SE)			
Women				
Fatigue	35 (1)	29 (2)	28 (2)	33 (1)
Sleep problems	29 (1)	27 (1)	28 (2)	28 (1)
Irritability	27 (1)	22 (1)	22 (2)	25 (1)
Worry	25 (1)	20 (1)	18 (2)	23 (1)
Depression	12 (1)	8 (1)	7 (1)	11 (1)
Depressive ideas	13 (1)	9 (1)	7 (1)	11 (1)
Anxiety	12 (1)	10 (1)	9 (1)	11 (1)
Obsessions	12 (1)	11 (1)	8 (2)	12 (1)
Concentration and forgetfulness	11 (1)	7 (1)	8 (2)	10 (1)
Somatic symptoms	11 (0)	7 (1)	9 (1)	10 (0)
Compulsions	8 (1)	7 (1)	5 (1)	8 (0)
Phobias	8 (0)	6 (1)	4 (1)	7 (0)
Worry about physical health	6 (0)	4 (1)	2 (1)	5 (0)
Panic	4 (0)	2 (0)	3 (1)	3 (0)
Base	*3263*	*1179*	*492*	*4933*
Men				
Fatigue	21 (1)	22 (1)	18 (2)	21 (1)
Sleep problems	21 (1)	22 (2)	16 (2)	21 (1)
Irritability	19 (1)	19 (1)	15 (2)	19 (1)
Worry	18 (1)	17 (1)	14 (2)	17 (1)
Depression	9 (1)	8 (1)	6 (1)	8 (0)
Depressive ideas	8 (1)	6 (1)	4 (1)	7 (0)
Anxiety	9 (1)	6 (1)	5 (1)	8 (0)
Obsessions	7 (1)	6 (1)	5 (1)	7 (0)
Concentration and forgetfulness	7 (0)	6 (1)	6 (1)	6 (0)
Somatic symptoms	5 (0)	5 (1)	4 (1)	5 (0)
Compulsions	5 (0)	5 (1)	4 (1)	5 (0)
Phobias	4 (0)	2 (0)	1 (0)	3 (0)
Worry about physical health	5 (0)	4 (1)	3 (1)	4 (0)
Panic	2 (0)	1 (0)	1 (0)	2 (0)
Base	*3187*	*1153*	*519*	*4859*
All adults				
Fatigue	28 (1)	26 (1)	23 (1)	27 (1)
Sleep problems	25 (1)	24 (1)	22 (2)	25 (1)
Irritability	23 (1)	20 (1)	18 (2)	22 (1)
Worry	21 (1)	18 (1)	16 (1)	20 (1)
Depression	10 (0)	8 (1)	6 (1)	10 (0)
Depressive ideas	10 (0)	8 (1)	5 (1)	9 (0)
Anxiety	10 (0)	8 (1)	7 (1)	10 (0)
Obsessions	10 (0)	9 (1)	7 (1)	9 (0)
Concentration and forgetfulness	9 (0)	7 (1)	7 (1)	8 (0)
Somatic symptoms	8 (0)	6 (1)	7 (1)	8 (0)
Compulsions	7 (0)	6 (1)	4 (1)	6 (0)
Phobias	6 (0)	4 (0)	3 (1)	5 (0)
Worry about physical health	5 (0)	4 (0)	2 (1)	5 (0)
Panic	3 (0)	2 (0)	2 (0)	2 (0)
Base	6450	2332	1010	9792

Table 5.13 Summary of significant odds ratios: CIS-R symptoms

Asterisks represent increases or decreases (shaded cells) in odds
For each variable, the reference group is the first category listed.

	Fatigue	Sleep problems	Irritability	Worry	Depression	Depressive ideas	Anxiety	Obsessions	Concentration forgetfulness	Somatic symptoms	Compulsions	Phobias	Worry/physical health	Panic
Sex:														
Male														
Female	**	**	**	**		**	**	**	**	**	**	**		**
Age:														
16-24														
25-34														
35-44			**			**				*			*	
45-54		*	**			**				**	*	*		
55-64			**	**	**	**			**		**	**		
Ethnicity:														
White														
West Indian/African					*									
Asian/Oriental			**										**	
Other														
Qualifications:														
A level or higher														
GCSE/O level												**	**	
Other				**								**		
None				**									**	
Family unit type:														
Couple/no children														
Couple: 1+ child		**	**					*			**		*	
Lone parent + child	**		*		**	**		*	*	*				
One person only	*	**	*	*	**	**	**	**	**	**		**		
Adult with parents	**							**					**	
Adult with one parent	**									*				
Employment status:														
Working full time														
Working part time			**					*			**			
Unemployed	**	**	**	**	**	**	**	**	**	**		**	**	**
Economically inactive	**	**	**	**	**	**	**	**	**	**	**	**	**	**
Occupation type:														
Non-manual														
Manual						*					**			
Accommodation:														
Detached														
Semi-detached					**									
Terraced			**				**						**	
Flat/maisonette							**						**	
Tenure:														
Owner/occupier														
Renter	**	**	*	**	**	**	**		**		**	**		**
Locality:														
Semi-rural/rural														
Urban	*		*	**	*	**				**		**		**

Table 5.14   Odds ratios of socio-demographic correlates of fatigue

		Adjusted OR	(95% CI)
Sex	**Male**	1.00	....
	Female	1.76**	(1.61-1.94)
Family unit type	**Couple, no children**	1.00	....
	Couple & child(ren)	1.09	(0.34-3.47)
	Lone parent & child(ren)	1.34**	(1.13-1.60)
	One person only	1.19*	(1.04-1.35)
	Adult with parents	0.64**	(0.51-0.80)
	Adult with one parent	0.62**	(0.45-0.85)
Tenure	**Owner-occupier**	1.00	....
	Renter	1.42**	(1.28-1.57)
Locality	**Semi-rural/rural**	1.00	....
	Urban	1.11*	(1.01-1.22)

Significance: *   p<0.05
             ** p<0.01

Table 5.15   Odds ratios of socio-demographic correlates of sleep problems

		Adjusted OR	(95% CI)
Sex	**Male**	1.00	....
	Female	1.32**	(1.18-1.46)
Age	**16-24**	1.00	....
	25-34	0.96	(0.80-1.15)
	35-44	1.16	(0.97-1.40)
	45-54	1.21*	(1.00-1.46)
	55-64	0.05	(0.86-1.27)
Family unit type	**Couple, no children**	1.00	....
	Couple & child(ren)	0.80**	(0.70-0.91)
	Lone parent & child(ren)	1.18	(0.98-1.42)
	One person only	1.24**	(1.09-1.42)
	Adult with parents	0.81	(0.63-1.04)
	Adult with one parent	0.75	(0.55-1.06)
Employment status	**Working full-time**	1.00	....
	Working part-time	1.33**	(1.16-1.54)
	Unemployed	1.85**	(1.56-2.18)
	Economically inactive	1.80**	(1.59-2.05)
Tenure	**Owner-occupier**	1.00	....
	Renter	1.16**	(1.04-1.29)

Significance: *   p<0.05
             ** p<0.01

Table 5.16 Odds ratios of socio-demographic correlates of irritability

		Adjusted OR	(95% CI)
Sex	**Male**	1.00	....
	Female	1.41**	(1.26-1.58)
Age	**16-24**	1.00	....
	25-34	0.88	(0.74-1.05)
	35-44	0.75**	(0.62-0.90)
	45-54	0.55**	(0.45-0.68)
	55-64	0.35**	(0.28-0.43)
Ethnicity	**White**	1.00	....
	West Indian or African	0.78	(0.53-1.14)
	Asian or Oriental	0.56**	(0.39-0.80)
	Other	0.89	(0.53-1.49)
Family unit type	**Couple, no children**	1.00	....
	Couple & child(ren)	1.37**	(1.19-1.58)
	Lone parent & child(ren)	1.26*	(1.03-1.54)
	One person only	0.84*	(0.71-0.98)
	Adult with parents	0.91	(0.70-1.17)
	Adult with one parent	0.76	(0.55-1.02)
Employment status	**Working full-time**	1.00	....
	Working part-time	1.05	(0.90-1.23)
	Unemployed	1.50**	(1.25-1.78)
	Economically inactive	1.35**	(1.17-1.55)
Accommodation	**Detached**	1.00	....
	Semi-detached	1.01	(0.86-1.17)
	Terraced	1.33**	(1.14-1.55)
	Flat or maisonette	1.15	(0.95-1.40)
Tenure	**Owner-occupier**	1.00	....
	Renter	1.14*	(1.01-1.29)
Locality	**Semi-rural/rural**	1.00	....
	Urban	1.13*	(1.01-1.27)

Significance: *   p<0.05
        ** p<0.01

Table 5.17   Odds ratios of socio-demographic correlates of worry

		Adjusted OR	(95% CI)
Sex	**Male**	1.00	....
	Female	1.42**	(1.26-1.60)
Age	**16-24**	1.00	....
	25-34	0.96	(0.81-1.15)
	35-44	1.13	(0.93-1.37)
	45-54	0.91	(0.75-1.12)
	55-64	0.63**	(0.51-0.78)
Family unit type	**Couple, no children**	1.00	....
	Couple & child(ren)	0.93	(0.81-1.07)
	Lone parent & child(ren)	1.19	(0.97-1.45)
	One person only	1.18*	(1.02-1.38)
	Adult with parents	0.81	(0.62-1.07)
	Adult with one parent	0.75	(0.53-1.04)
Employment status	**Working full-time**	1.00	....
	Working part-time	0.97	(0.83-1.14)
	Unemployed	1.67**	(1.40-1.99)
	Economically inactive	1.20**	(1.05-1.39)
Accommodation	**Detached**	1.00	....
	Semi-detached	0.81**	(0.69-0.94)
	Terraced	0.98	(0.84-1.15)
	Flat or maisonette	1.04	(0.86-1.25)
Tenure	**Owner-occupier**	1.00	....
	Renter	1.20**	(1.06-1.36)
Locality	**Semi-rural/rural**	1.00	....
	Urban	1.18**	(1.04-1.32)

Significance: *   p<0.05
             ** p<0.01

Table 5.18 Odds ratios of socio-demographic correlates of depression

		Adjusted OR	(95%CI)
Age	16-24	1.00	....
	25-34	1.07	(0.83-1.36)
	35-44	1.23	(0.96-1.59)
	45-54	0.67**	(0.88-1.50)
	55-64	0.67**	(0.50-0.90
Ethnicity	White	1.00	....
	West Indian or African	1.67*	(1.10-2.51)
	Asian or Oriental	1.15	(0.76-1.74)
	Other	1.74	(0.97-3.09)
Qualification	A level or higher	1.00	....
	GCSE/O level	1.10	(0.91-1.34)
	Other	1.38**	(1.09-1.75)
	None	1.44**	(1.20-1.74)
Family unit type	Couple, no children	1.00	....
	Couple & child(ren)	1.05	(0.86-1.28)
	Lone parent & child(ren)	1.45**	(1.12-1.90)
	One person only	1.49**	(1.21-1.82)
	Adult with parents	1.16	(0.81-1.66)
	Adult with one parent	1.13	(0.74-1.72)
Employment status	Working full-time	1.00	....
	Working part-time	1.20	(0.98-1.49)
	Unemployed	2.14**	(1.72-2.65)
	Economically Inactive	1.80**	(1.51-2.15)
Tenure	Owner occupier	1.00	....
	Renter	1.29**	(1.10-1.51)
Locality	Semi-rural/rural	1.00	....
	Urban	1.19*	(1.02-1.39)

Significance: * p<0.05

            ** p<0.01

Table 5.19   Odds ratios of socio-demographic correlates of depressive ideas

		Adjusted OR	(95% CI)
Sex	**Male**	1.00	....
	Female	1.53**	(1.30-1.80)
Age	**16-24**	1.00	....
	25-34	0.93	(0.73-1.19)
	35-44	1.12	(0.87-1.44)
	45-54	1.09	(0.84-1.42)
	55-64	0.56**	(0.42-0.75)
Ethnicity	**White**	1.00	....
	West Indian or African	1.49	(0.98-2.26)
	Asian or Oriental	1.33	(0.89-2.00)
	Other	1.71	(0.96-3.07)
Family unit type	**Couple, no children**	1.00	....
	Couple & child(ren)	1.00	(0.81-1.25)
	Lone parent & child(ren)	1.78**	(1.38-2.30)
	One person only	1.55**	(1.25-1.93)
	Adult with parents	1.10	(0.76-1.59)
	Adult with one parent	1.00	(0.64-1.58)
Employment status	**Working full-time**	1.00	....
	Working part-time	1.30*	(1.06-1.63)
	Unemployed	2.66**	(2.14-3.32)
	Economically inactive	1.77**	(1.46-2.14)
Occupation type	**Non manual**	1.00	....
	Manual	1.17*	(1.01-1.35)
Tenure	**Owner-occupier**	1.00	....
	Renter	1.41**	(1.20-1.66)
Locality	**Semi-rural/rural**	1.00	....
	Urban	1.25**	(1.06-1.46)

Significance: * $p < 0.05$
              ** $p < 0.01$

Table 5.20   Odds ratios of socio-demographic correlates of anxiety

		Adjusted OR	(95% CI)
Sex	**Male**	1.00	....
	Female	1.31**	(1.12-1.53)
Age	**16-24**	1.00	....
	25-34	1.30	(1.00-1.69)
	35-44	1.61**	(1.22-2.11)
	45-54	1.86**	(1.41-2.45)
	55-64	1.25	(0.93-1.67)
Family unit type	**Couple, no children**	1.00	....
	Couple & child(ren)	1.01	(0.83-1.22)
	Lone parent & child(ren)	1.27	(0.99-1.64)
	One person only	1.31**	(1.08-1.59)
	Adult with parents	1.01	(0.68-1.50)
	Adult with one parent	0.85	(0.53-1.37)
Employment status	**Working full-time**	1.00	....
	Working part-time	1.00	(0.80-1.25)
	Unemployed	1.98**	(1.59-2.45)
	Economically inactive	1.75**	(1.47 2.09)
Accommodation	**Detached**	1.00	....
	Semi-detached	1.15	(1.93-1.43)
	Terraced	1.37**	(1.10-1.69)
	Flat or maisonette	1.52**	(1.18-1.96)
Tenure	**Owner-occupier**	1.00	....
	Renter	1.43**	(1.22-1.68)

Significance: * $p<0.05$

      ** $p<0.01$

Table 5.21   Odds ratios of socio-demographic correlates of obsessions

		Adjusted OR	(95% CI)
Sex	Male	1.00	....
	Female	1.64**	(1.40-1.92)
Age	16-24	1.00	....
	25-34	0.90	(0.71-1.14)
	35-44	1.02	(0.79-1.32)
	45-54	0.83	(0.65-1.08)
	55-64	0.52**	(0.39-0.68)
Family unit type	Couple, no children	1.00	....
	Couple & child(ren)	0.79*	(0.64-0.96)
	Lone parent & child(ren)	1.33*	(1.04-1.72)
	One person only	1.48**	(1.22-1.79)
	Adult with parents	0.57**	(0.39-0.85)
	Adult with one parent	0.84	(0.54-1.32)
Employment status	Working full-time	1.00	....
	Working part-time	1.25*	(1.01-1.56)
	Unemployed	2.51**	(2.02-3.11)
	Economically inactive	1.58**	(1.32-1.90)

Significance: *   p<0.05
              ** p<0.01

Table 5.22   Odds ratios of socio-demographic correlates of concentration and forgetfulness

		Adjusted OR	(95% CI)
Sex	Male	1.00	....
	Female	1.34**	(1.14-1.58)
Age	16-24	1.00	....
	25-34	0.98	(0.75-1.28)
	35-44	1.12	(0.85-1.48)
	45-54	1.23	(0.94-1.63)
	55-64	0.75	(0.56-1.01)
Family unit type	Couple, no children	1.00	....
	Couple & child(ren)	1.11	(0.90-1.38)
	Lone parent & child(ren)	1.41*	(1.06-1.87)
	One person only	1.80**	(1.46-2.22)
	Adult with parents	0.70	(0.45-1.09)
	Adult with one parent	1.00	(0.61-1.63)
Employment status	Working full-time	1.00	....
	Working part-time	1.11	(0.89-1.40)
	Unemployed	1.66**	(1.30-2.13)
	Economically inactive	1.78**	(1.47-2.15)
Tenure	Owner-occupier	1.00	....
	Renter	1.24**	(1.06-1.46)

Significance: *   p<0.05
              ** p<0.01

Table 5.23   Odds ratios of socio-demographic correlates of somatic symptoms

		Adjusted OR	(95% CI)
Sex	Male	1.00	....
	Female	1.73**	(1.46-2.06)
Age	16-24	1.00	....
	25-34	1.07	(0.79-1.44)
	35-44	1.42*	(1.04-1.93)
	45-54	1.69**	(1.24-2.29)
	55-64	1.06	(0.77-1.46)
Family unit type	Couple, no children	1.00	....
	Couple & child(ren)	1.09	(0.88-1.35)
	Lone parent & child(ren)	1.41*	(1.07-1.86)
	One person only	1.39**	(1.13-1.73)
	Adult with parents	0.67	(0.41-1.09)
	Adult with one parent	0.48*	(0.24-0.96)
Employment status	Working full-time	1.00	....
	Working part-time	1.04	(0.83-1.31)
	Unemployed	1.51**	(1.16-1.98)
	Economically inactive	1.53**	(1.26-1.86)
Locality	Semi-rural/rural	1.00	....
	Urban	1.24**	(1.05-1.47)

Significance: *   p<0.05
           ** p<0.01

Table 5.24   Odds ratios of socio-demographic correlates of compulsions

		Adjusted OR	(95% CI)
Sex	Male	1.00	....
	Female	1.32**	(1.10-1.60)
Age	16-24	1.00	....
	25-34	0.84	(0.64-1.11)
	35-44	0.77	(0.57-1.04)
	45-54	0.67*	(0.50-0.91)
	55-64	0.53**	(0.39-0.73)
Family unit type	Couple, no children	1.00	....
	Couple & child(ren)	0.70**	(0.55-0.89)
	Lone parent & child(ren)	1.14	(0.83-1.56)
	One person only	1.25	(0.99-1.59)
	Adult with parents	0.73	(0.47-1.12)
	Adult with one parent	1.22	(0.77-1.91)
Employment status	Working full-time	1.00	....
	Working part-time	1.40**	(1.09-1.81)
	Unemployed	1.25	(0.93-1.67)
	Economically inactive	1.48**	(1.19-1.83)
Occupation type	Non manual	1.00	....
	Manual	1.26**	(1.06-1.49)
Tenure	Owner-occupier	1.00	....
	Renter	1.28**	(1.06-1.55)

Significance: *   p<0.05
           ** p<0.01

Table 5.25   Odds ratios of socio-demographic correlates of phobic symptoms

		Adjusted OR	(95% CI)
Sex	Male	1.00	....
	Female	2.07**	(1.67-2.57)
Age	16-24	1.00	....
	25-34	0.93	(0.70-1.25)
	35-44	1.00	(0.73-1.37)
	45-54	0.68*	(0.48-0.96)
	55-64	0.56**	(0.39-0.81)
Qualifications	A level or higher	1.00	....
	GCSE/ O level	1.45**	(1.12-1.87)
	Other	1.50**	(1.10-2.06)
	None	1.27	(0.99-1.64)
Family unit type	Couple, no children	1.00	....
	Couple & child(ren)	0.89	(0.68-1.18)
	Lone parent & child(ren)	1.11	(0.78-1.59)
	One person only	1.55**	(1.18-2.04)
	Adult with parents	1.29	(0.82-2.00)
	Adult with one parent	1.32	(0.78-2.21)
Employment status	Working full-time	1.00	....
	Working part-time	0.85	(0.64-1.14)
	Unemployed	1.93**	(1.44-2.60)
	Economically inactive	1.67**	(1.32-2.11)
Tenure	Owner-occupier	1.00	....
	Renter	1.42**	(1.17-1.73)
Locality	Semi-rural/rural	1.00	....
	Urban	1.41**	(1.13-1.74)

Significance: * $p<0.05$
             ** $p<0.01$

Table 5.26   Odds ratios of socio-demographic correlates of worry about physical health

		Adjusted OR	(95% CI)
Age	**16-24**	1.00	....
	25-34	1.10	(0.76-1.59)
	35-44	1.63*	(1.12-2.37)
	45-54	1.45	(0.98-2.13)
	55-64	0.92	(0.61-1.38)
Ethnicity	**White**	1.00	....
	West Indian or African	1.38	(0.77-2.48)
	Asian or Oriental	1.94**	(1.21-3.10)
	Other	0.41	(0.10-1.67)
Qualifications	**A level or higher**	1.00	....
	GCSE/ O level	1.45**	(1.10-1.90)
	Other	1.07	(0.75-1.53)
	None	1.47**	(1.13-1.89)
Family unit type	**Couple, no children**	1.00	....
	Couple & child(ren)	0.75*	(0.57-0.98)
	Lone parent & child(ren)	0.78	(0.54-1.13)
	One person only	1.12	(0.87-1.44)
	Adult with parents	0.37**	(0.19-0.73)
	Adult with one parent	0.57	(0.29-1.12)
Employment status	**Working full-time**	1.00	....
	Working part-time	1.06	(0.77-1.45)
	Unemployed	1.97**	(1.44-2.70)
	Economically inactive	2.58**	(2.04-3.27)
Accommodation	**Detached**	1.00	....
	Semi-detached	1.17	(0.86-1.61)
	Terraced	1.60**	(1.17-2.19)
	Flat or maisonette	1.91**	(1.37-2.67)

Significance: * p<0.05 ** p<0.01

Table 5.27 Odds ratios of socio-demographic correlates of panic

		Adjusted OR	(95% CI)
Sex	**Male**	1.00	....
	Female	1.74**	(1.30-2.35)
Age	**16-24**	1.00	....
	25-34	1.07	(0.72-1.59)
	35-44	1.28	(0.85-1.94)
	45-54	1.28	(0.83-1.98)
	55-64	0.64	(0.40-1.03)
Employment status	**Working full-time**	1.00	....
	Working part-time	0.92	(0.60-1.41)
	Unemployed	1.87**	(1.22-2.89)
	Economically inactive	2.21**	(1.59-3.05)
Tenure	**Owner-occupier**	1.00	....
	Renter	1.95**	(1.49-2.57)
Locality	**Semi-rural/rural**	1.00	....
	Urban	1.72**	(1.27-2.37)

Significance: * p<0.05 ** p<0.01

6 Prevalence of psychiatric disorders

6.1 Introduction

This chapter reports on the prevalence rates of the neurotic disorders, functional psychoses, and alcohol and drug dependence. Odds ratios are also presented summarising the effects of the socio-demographic variables on the odds of having each disorder.

Assessing the prevalence of neurotic disorders

The prevalence of neurotic disorders was based on the presence, frequency, severity and duration of various symptoms as reported by subjects in the revised Clinical Interview Schedule (CIS-R).[1] See Chapter 2, section 2.1 for more information.

Six neurotic disorders were identified:

- depressive episode including all levels of depression (mild, moderate and severe)
- phobias, encompassing agoraphobia, social phobia and specific isolated phobias
- obsessive compulsive disorder
- panic disorder
- generalised anxiety disorder
- mixed anxiety and depressive disorder, a 'catch all'category which included people with significant neurotic psychopathology who could not be coded into any of the other five neurotic disorders

The disorders were organised hierarchically. This meant that when an individual was diagnosed as having more than one disorder the 'highest' disorder assumed precedence, and the person received that single diagnosis. The algorithms for the creation of these categories of disorder are included in Appendix B, Part 2.

Prevalence rates for neurotic disorders are shown as rates per thousand population in the past week; that is, where the informant had experienced relevant symptoms of the disorder in the past week. As a result of rounding and weighting the rate of any neurotic disorder may not exactly equal the sum of the rates of individual disorders.

Assessing prevalence rates of functional psychosis

Two stages were involved in obtaining prevalence rates of psychosis: sifting (carried out by OPCS interviewers) and assessment (made by clinicians).

The OPCS sift comprised four elements:

A psychosis screening questionnaire (PSQ) covered the experience of mania, thought disorder, paranoia, delusions and auditory hallucinations in the past year.[2]

Respondents were also asked whether..

- they suffered from a psychotic illness,
- they had been told by their doctor that they suffered from a psychotic illness, or
- reported that they were currently taking any prescribed anti-psychotic medication.

Individuals who sifted positive for psychosis on one or more of the above criteria had a SCAN follow-up interview.[3] Where it was not possible to carry out a clinical interview, (because of refusals or non-contacts), the OPCS sift data was re-examined taking into account the analysis of the relationship between sift and assessment data for the successful interviews. Those taking anti-psychotic medication (tablets or depot injections) and who also reported that they had a psychotic illness and/or that their doctor had told them that they had a psychotic illness were regarded as having a functional psychosis.

Assessing alcohol and drug dependence

Questions relating to alcohol and drug dependence were included in a self-completion questionnaire (Appendix C) administered to all informants whether or not they came up as having a mental health problem on the assessment schedules.

The twelve questions on alcohol dependence were taken from the National Alcohol Survey carried out in the USA in 1984. An anglicised version was created to measure the three components of dependence: loss of control, symptomatic behaviour and binge drinking.

Questions on drug use and dependence were taken from the ECA study.[4] In this study informants were shown a list of ten types of drug (with examples of their most common names) and were asked questions on use, dependence and problems by referring to this list.

6.2 Distribution of psychiatric disorders by personal characteristics

About one in six adults, aged 16 to 64, in Great Britain suffered a neurotic disorder in the week before interview *(Figure 6.1)*. The most prevalent neurotic disorder was mixed anxiety and depressive disorder (77 cases per thousand). Further analysis showed that 66% of those with a diagnosis of mixed anxiety and depression reported CIS-R symptoms of either depression, depressive ideas, or anxiety. The remaining 35% reported CIS-R symptoms of fatigue, sleep, irritability or worry. Generalised anxiety was found in 31 adults per thousand; the remaining disorders (phobias, depressive episode, Obsessive-Compulsive Disorder, and panic) were less prevalent, ranging from 21 to 8 cases per thousand.

For all six neurotic disorders the prevalence was higher among women than men. The difference between the rates for women and men was greatest for mixed anxiety and depressive disorder (99 and 54 cases per thousand respectively).

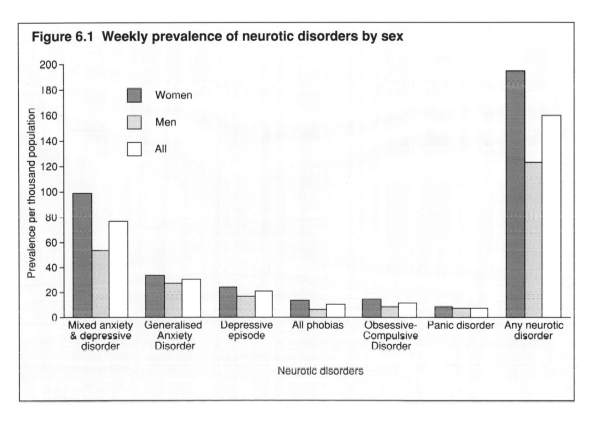

Figure 6.1 Weekly prevalence of neurotic disorders by sex

Functional psychosis (schizophrenia, manic depressive psychosis and schizo-affective disorder) had a yearly prevalence rate of 4 per thousand; the same proportion was found among men and women *(Figure 6.2)*.

Differences in the overall yearly prevalence rate of alcohol and drug dependence by sex were in the opposite direction to those found for neurotic disorders: men were three times more likely than women to have alcohol dependence and twice as likely to be drug dependent *(Figure 6.2)*.

Age

The overall prevalence of any neurotic disorder showed some variation by age although differences did not reach statistical significance. Rates appeared lowest at the extremes of the distribution; 126 per thousand among those aged 16-19 and 133 per thousand among 60-64 year olds. The highest rates of over 170 per thousand were found in the centre of the distribution. In each age group the prevalence of any neurotic disorder was higher among women than among men.

The trends found for individual disorders varied. Mixed anxiety and depressive disorder increased with age, peaking in the 30-34 age group and declining thereafter. Generalised Anxiety Disorder showed different patterns among men and women; for both sexes this disorder initially increased with age, however among men the prevalence reached a maximum among 40-44 year olds and fell among older men. For women the peak came in the oldest age group, with prevalence higher among the over 50s than among younger women. There was no apparent trend in the prevalence of depressive episode or panic disorder by age. For both men and women, Obsessive Compulsive Disorder was at a maximum among 20-24 year olds. Phobias were most prevalent among the youngest group with a prevalence of 24 per thousand. Among other age groups phobias were fairly consistent affecting around 11 per thousand.

The prevalence of functional psychoses showed no obvious patterns, with only small differences in prevalence among the age

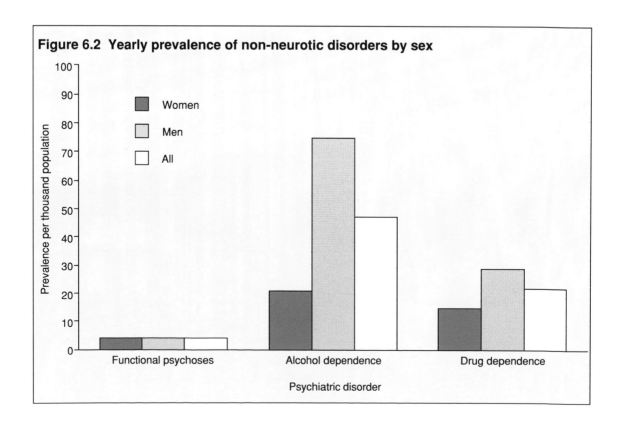

Figure 6.2 Yearly prevalence of non-neurotic disorders by sex

groups. Because of the relatively small overall yearly prevalence of 4 per thousand, and large standard errors, interpretation of small differences are difficult. However, the highest prevalence of functional psychosis in women was observed in the 30-34 year old age group, and for men was observed between the ages of 55 and 64 years.

The highest prevalence of alcohol and drug dependence was found among young adults, aged 16 to 24, particularly young men, aged 20-24, with a yearly prevalence of 176 per thousand for alcohol dependence and 111 per thousand for drug dependence. *(Table 6.1)*

Ethnicity

As stated in Chapters 4 and 5, ethnic differences were difficult to interpret because of the small numbers in the sample who regarded themselves as belonging to minority ethnic groups. The same cautions about small bases apply to the distribution of psychiatric disorders by ethnicity. When analysed by sex the bases were smaller still, making the differences between distributions correspondingly more difficult to interpret. The presence of any neurotic disorder appeared to be higher among women than among men in every ethnic group, with the highest rate of psychosis observed among West Indian or African women. However, none of these observed differences were statistically significant. *(Table 6.2)*

Marital status

The prevalence of every neurotic disorder varied markedly with marital status for both men and women. The rates of any neurotic disorder among women were highest among the divorced (304 per thousand) and lowest among the married (170 per thousand), while among men the highest rates were among the separated (309 per thousand) and lowest among the married and cohabiting (116 and 115 per thousand respectively).

Among men, those who were separated had the highest rates of mixed anxiety and depressive

disorder, depressive episode, phobias and Obsessive Compulsive Disorder. In the case of depressive episode, the rate among separated men (111 per thousand) was almost eight times the rate in married men (14 per thousand) and ten times that for cohabiting men (11 per thousand).

For women the separated group also had the highest prevalence of depressive episode, although at 56 cases per thousand the rate was half that for men of the same marital status. The highest rates of the other disorders were mostly found in the widowed or divorced groups.

There was a clear relationship between being separated or divorced and having a psychotic illness. The rate of functional psychoses was highest in women in the divorced group (15 per thousand) while among men it was highest in the widowed group (23 per thousand). Alcohol and drug dependence were most prevalent among single people, though further analysis suggested that this finding represents an age effect — over 75% of single people were aged under 29. Alcohol dependence was clearly most prevalent among single and separated men, while alcohol dependence among women was highest among single people. These patterns were also found for drug dependence. *(Table 6.3)*

Education

There was little apparent pattern to the distribution of the individual disorders by age when finished full-time education, both for men and for women. The prevalence of any neurotic disorder was highest in men and women who finished full-time education aged 14 or under, or at age 15.

Similarly, while there was no obvious pattern to the prevalence of individual disorders by educational qualifications, the prevalence of any neurotic disorder was highest for men and women with no qualifications (145 and 224 per thousand respectively). This group however had the lowest levels of alcohol dependence, probably reflecting the fact that they were also the oldest age group — over 40% of this group were aged 50 or over.

For both sexes, the prevalence of functional psychoses was highest among those with GCE 'A' levels or higher qualifications (men, 10 per thousand; women, 8 per thousand).

For women, alcohol and drug dependence were most prevalent among students, (i.e. those not yet finished full-time education) with 82 cases per thousand and 50 cases per thousand respectively. Among men, alcohol dependence was highest among those who finished full-time education at 16 (101 per thousand), with the next highest prevalence found among students (78 per thousand). The highest prevalence of drug dependence among men was also found in the student group (80 per thousand).*(Tables 6.4 and 6.5)*

Employment status

Employment status is a major factor in understanding the differences in prevalence rates of all psychiatric disorders in adults. About one quarter of unemployed people had exhibited a neurotic disorder in the past week compared with about 1 in 8 of those working full time.

Looking at specific disorders among women, the highest rates of every neurotic disorder except panic disorder were found in the unemployed group. For example, the rate of depressive episode was over five times higher in this group than among women working full time, and the rates for all other neurotic disorders except panic disorder were at least twice as high.

Among men, it also appeared that those working full time had the lowest rates of most neurotic disorders. The prevalence of any neurotic disorder among men in this employment group was approximately half the rate found among the unemployed and the economically inactive.

The rate of functional psychoses was highest (at 14 per thousand) among men who were economically

inactive, i.e. not working and not seeking work, and again was lowest among those working full time. For women, the highest rate was found among the unemployed at 10 per thousand.

Drug dependence among women was much higher among the unemployed group than among any other (55 per thousand) and much lower among the full-time employed (7 per thousand). Among men, alcohol and drug dependence were both much higher among the unemployed group (117 and 96 per thousand respectively). *(Table 6.6)*

Social class

There were some differences in psychiatric morbidity by social class. Among women, the lowest rates of any neurotic disorder were found in Social Classes I and II, and the highest in Social Classes IV and V. Variations were less marked for men, although the lowest rate of any neurotic disorder appearing in Social Class I (60 per thousand) was far lower.

Functional psychoses also showed a relationship with social class, with the highest prevalence of psychosis in both men and women found in Social Class V (17 and 16 per thousand respectively). Alcohol and drug dependence fit in with the general pattern, with high rates of alcohol and drug dependence found among those in Social Class V. *(Table 6.7)*

6.3 Distribution of psychiatric disorders by family characteristics

Family unit type

Strong variations in the prevalence of psychiatric morbidity emerged when the disorders were examined by family unit type. The prevalence of any neurotic disorder was highest among lone parents (281 cases per thousand) and lowest among adults living with their parents (112 per thousand). Couples with no children also had low prevalence of any neurotic disorders (134 per thousand) while those in one-person family units had the second highest rates of neurosis (209 per thousand). The same patterns were found for men and women.

The prevalence of all individual disorders except Generalised Anxiety Disorder was highest in the lone parent group.

Among women, the rate of functional psychosis was highest among lone parents, and among men the highest rate was found among those living alone.

Alcohol dependence was highest for men among those living alone, while in women alcohol dependence was highest among adults living with one parent. The higher prevalence of alcohol dependence in these family unit types is likely to be due to the higher proportion of younger people living in these circumstances; for example, as noted above (Table 6.1) alcohol dependence was particularly prevalent among men aged under 35, and around half of those living alone were in this age group. Similarly for women, alcohol dependence was particularly prevalent among those aged under 40, and further analysis showed that the majority of women living with one parent were below this age.

Drug dependence was highest among adults living with one parent, both for men and for women. *(Table 6.8)*

6.4 Distribution of psychiatric disorders by household characteristics

Tenure

The prevalence of the whole range of neurotic disorders was generally higher among those living in rented accommodation than among owner occupiers. Overall the rate of any neurotic disorder for those renting from Housing Associations or Local Authorities was 244 per thousand compared with rates of 125 and 138 per thousand among those owning their homes outright or with a mortgage.

There were very substantial differences between owner occupiers and renters in the prevalence of psychosis, alcohol and drug dependence. Among men the rate of psychosis, alcohol and drug dependence was three times higher among renters than among those who owned their property outright or had a mortgage. Among women, the rate of psychosis was approximately five times greater among those renting their accommodation. *(Table 6.9)*

Type of accommodation

The overall rate of neurosis was highest among those living in flats and maisonettes, 221 per thousand, and lowest among those in detached or semi-detached houses (123 and 137 cases per thousand respectively). For both men and women the highest rate of functional psychoses was found among those living in flats or maisonettes: 8 per thousand among both men and women in this type of accommodation. *(Table 6.10)*

6.5 Prevalence of psychiatric disorders by region and locality

Country and Region

Overall there was very little difference in the prevalence of any neurotic disorder in England, Scotland and Wales. Among men however, there was an apparent, yet not statistically significant, difference in Wales where rates of depressive episode were higher than in the other countries while rates of mixed anxiety and depression were lower.

There were wide variations between the Regional Health Authorities (RHAs) of England[5] in the prevalence of neurotic disorders although many of these were not found to be statistically significant. Variations partly reflect the differences shown above in personal, family and household characteristics.

The highest prevalences of 'any neurotic disorder' were found in Mersey and North East Thames, both with rates above 200 per thousand. The lowest rates of below 130 per thousand were found among those in Wessex and the South Western RHA.

The overall prevalence of the functional psychoses varied from 2 per thousand in Trent and in North East Thames to 9 per thousand in South East Thames. However, it should be emphasised that the low numbers in each category made it difficult to draw firm conclusions about regional differences in the prevalence of psychosis. This was particularly true when the data were analysed by sex: examination of the sampling errors shows that the Regions' confidence intervals overlap, indicating no significant difference between them. *(Table 6.11)*

Locality

A major trend was identified when psychiatric morbidity was examined by locality. The prevalence of Generalised Anxiety Disorder, depressive episode, phobias, psychosis, alcohol and drug dependence was overall approximately twice as high in urban as in rural populations. This pattern was apparent for both sexes. For women, the prevalence of drug dependence in rural areas was particularly low at 2 per thousand, compared to 18 and 12 per thousand in urban and semi-rural areas. The prevalence of drug dependence among men in rural areas was around half that in urban areas (16 compared with 34 per thousand). The lower prevalence of these disorders in rural areas may again represent an age effect: Table 6.1 showed that the prevalence of drug and alcohol dependence was highest among those aged under 35, and further analysis of the data showed the proportion of individuals in this age group to be significantly higher in urban than in rural areas (47.3% compared with 33.7%, p<0.01). *(Table 6.12)*

6.6 Odds ratios of socio-demographic correlates of psychiatric disorders

Multiple logistic regression was used to produce odds ratios for the socio-demographic correlates

of each of the main categories of psychiatric disorder. Each disorder was coded as a dichotomous variable indicating the presence or absence of the disorder. Mild, moderate and severe depressive episode were grouped into one psychiatric disorder category, 'depressive episode' as indicated in *Table 6.14*.

Table 6.13 is a summary table of all significant odds ratios, indicating the socio-demographic variables which were found to influence the odds of having any disorder. Tables 6.14 to 6.22 show the socio-demographic correlates with significant odds ratios for each of the neurotic disorders, for functional psychosis, and for alcohol and drug dependence. Several variables are shown as significant in more than one table, indicating that the presence of these variables significantly increased the odds of having those disorders.

From Table 6.13, two variables appear to be strongly related to the psychiatric disorders. The first variable, employment status, significantly increased the odds of depressive episode, phobia, Obsessive Compulsive Disorder, Generalised Anxiety Disorder, mixed anxiety and depressive disorder, functional psychoses and drug dependence. The second variable, age group, significantly affected the odds of five disorders (Obsessive Compulsive Disorder, Generalised Anxiety Disorder, mixed anxiety and depressive disorder, alcohol dependence, drug dependence) as did the variable tenure (panic disorder, Generalised Anxiety Disorder, mixed anxiety and depressive disorder, functional psychoses, drug dependence).

Examination of employment status in Tables 6.14 to 6.22 shows that the odds of having most disorders were increased by being in the unemployed group. The same increase was observed for the economically inactive group. With respect to age, there is a clear trend of decreasing alcohol and drug dependence with increasing age. In terms of family unit type, being a lone parent compared with being in a couple increased the odds of three disorders (depressive episode, mixed anxiety and depressive disorder, alcohol dependence), while living alone increased the odds of depressive episode, mixed anxiety and depressive disorder and both alcohol and drug dependence.

Tenure, (being a renter rather than an owner-occupier) significantly increased the odds of panic disorder, Generalised Anxiety Disorder, mixed anxiety and depressive disorder, functional psychoses and drug dependence.

Being female increased the odds of two disorders (Generalised Anxiety Disorder, mixed anxiety and depressive disorder) and decreased the odds of two disorders (alcohol and drug dependence). Urban residence increased the odds of three disorders (phobia, depressive episode, Generalised Anxiety Disorder).

The association between the socio-demographic variables and psychiatric disorders are examined in more detail in the following sections.

Sex

The odds of two disorders were increased by being female. The odds of Generalised Anxiety Disorder were increased by about a third (OR=1.31) and the odds of mixed anxiety and depressive disorder were increased by more than two thirds (OR=1.73). The odds of alcohol and drug dependence on the other hand were significantly decreased by being female (ORs=0.26, 0.64).

The odds of depressive episode were not affected by sex when all other socio-demographic factors were controlled for. The odds of depressive symptoms assessed by the CIS-R had similarly been found to be unrelated to sex (see Chapter 5).

Age

Age was associated with the odds of most disorders. As expected, the odds of both alcohol and drug dependence decreased with increasing age compared with the reference group (age 16-24). The odds of mixed anxiety and depressive disorder and Obsessive Compulsive Disorder

were decreased by being in the oldest age group, while the odds of Generalised Anxiety Disorder appeared to increase with increasing age.

Ethnicity

Ethnicity was significantly related to the odds of two disorders. The odds of alcohol dependence were considerably decreased by being in the Asian or Oriental group compared with the reference group (White). The odds of phobia were more than doubled by being in the Asian or Oriental group (OR=2.34).

Qualifications

Having no qualifications increased the odds of depressive episode (OR=1.67).

Family unit type

Several categories within this variable affected the odds of psychiatric disorder. Compared with a couple with no children (the reference group), living alone significantly increased the odds of four disorders. The largest increase in odds related to drug dependency, the odds of which it almost trebled (OR=2.95). The odds of depressive episode and alcohol dependency were more than doubled by being in this family unit type, (ORs=2.32, 2.08) and the odds of mixed anxiety and depressive disorder were also significantly increased (OR=1.47).

The odds of three disorders were significantly increased by being a lone parent with a child, compared with the reference group (couple, no children), with the odds of depressive episode being more than doubled (OR=2.60). The odds of alcohol dependence were increased by more than two thirds, and the odds of mixed anxiety and depressive disorder were increased by about half (OR=1.48).

For the group 'adult living with one parent' there was no change in the odds of the neurotic disorders or of functional psychosis compared with the reference group (couple, no children). However the odds of drug dependence were more than doubled (OR=2.43) and the odds of alcohol dependence were increased by 79%.

Employment status

Unemployment significantly increased the odds of seven disorders compared with the reference group (working full time). It almost quadrupled the odds of drug dependence (OR=3.80) after controlling for other socio-demographic variables. Unemployment also approximately trebled the odds of phobia (OR=3.11) and functional psychosis (OR=2.98). It more than doubled the odds of depressive episode (OR=2.66), Generalised Anxiety Disorder (OR=2.19) and Obsessive Compulsive Disorder (OR=2.11) and increased the odds of mixed anxiety and depressive disorder by more than two-thirds (OR=1.73).

Being economically inactive increased the odds of functional psychosis and phobia (ORs=3.46, 3.28). It also increased the odds of depressive episode, drug dependence, Obsessive Compulsive Disorder and Generalised Anxiety Disorder (ORs=2.87, 2.34, 2.04, 1.44).

Accommodation

Type of accommodation was found to be related to two disorders, alcohol dependence and drug dependence. The odds of both these disorders were increased by living in either terraced housing or a flat or maisonette compared with the reference group (detached accommodation).

Tenure

Living in rented accommodation compared with being an owner-occupier greatly increased the odds of functional psychosis (OR=4.00) and more than doubled the odds of panic disorder (OR=2.46). It also increased the odds of drug dependence by about a half (OR=1.57). The odds of Generalised Anxiety Disorder and mixed anxiety and depressive disorder were also increased (ORs=1.42, 1.22).

Locality

The odds of phobia, depressive episode and Generalised Anxiety Disorder were significantly increased among those living in an urban area compared with an urban or semi-rural area (ORs=1.66, 1.38, 1.30). *(Tables 6.14-6.22)*

6.7 Odds ratios for the co-occurrence of psychiatric disorders

Odds ratios were also calculated to estimate the extent of comorbidity between psychiatric disorders. This shows the increased odds of having a second comorbid disorder for each psychiatric disorder. In order to do this the hierarchical rules relating to the disorders were abandoned.

Table 6.23 shows these odds ratios for all cases. In common with the methods used in the ECA study [4] odds ratios were taken to be significant when the ratio exceeded 10.00 and the lower bound of the confidence interval exceeded 4.00, and only significant odds ratios have been tabulated.

Among all cases, Obsessive Compulsive Disorder was significantly associated with three disorders: depression, phobia and Generalised Anxiety Disorder.

Generalised Anxiety Disorder occurs twice in Table 6.23. As well as its association with Obsessive Compulsive Disorder, GAD was significantly associated with depression. *(Table 6.23)*

Notes and references

1. Lewis, G., Pelosi, A.J. and Dunn, G. (1992). Measuring psychiatric disorder in the community: a standardised assessment for use by lay interviewers. *Psychological Medicine*, **22**, 465-486.

2. Bebbington, P.E. and Nayani, T. (1995). The Psychosis Screening Questionnaire, in *International Journal of Methods in Psychiatric Research.* **5**: 11-19

3. Wing, J.K., Babor, T., Brugha, T., Burke, J., Cooper, J.E., Giel, R., Jablensky,A., Regier, D., and Sartorius, N. (1990). SCAN:Schedules for clinical assessment in neuropsychiatry. *Archives of General Psychiatry*, **47**, 586-593.

4   Robins, L.N. and Regier, D.A. (eds) (1991). *Psychiatric disorders in America: the Epidemiological Catchment Area Study.* The Free Press (Macmillan Inc.), New York.

5. On 1st April 1994 the 14 NHS regions were replaced by eight regions. At the time the survey took place however, the 14 regions were still in existence and this is reflected in the relevant tables.

Table 6.1 Prevalence of psychiatric disorders by age and sex(rate per thousand population)

	Age										All
	16-19	20-24	25-29	30-34	35-39	40-44	45-49	50-54	55-59	60-64	
Women *Rate per thousand in past week(SE)*											
Mixed anxiety and depressive disorder	87 (20)	111 (14)	105 (12)	122 (13)	115(13)	110(14)	108(13)	92 (15)	49 (11)	55(10)	99 (5)
GAD	4 (5)	23 (7)	22 (6)	26 (7)	31 (8)	35(9)	39 (8)	61 (12)	47 (10)	64(11)	34 (3)
Depressive episode	32 (12)	26 (7)	23 (6)	35 (7)	23 (6)	27(7)	31 (8)	22 (7)	18 (6)	5 (2)	25 (2)
All phobias	45 (14)	14 (5)	11 (4)	15 (5)	18 (5)	8(5)	13 (5)	10 (5)	11 (4)	6 (2)	14 (2)
OCD	12 (8)	29 (8)	13 (4)	9 (5)	13 (5)	16(6)	8 (4)	18 (6)	20 (7)	4 (2)	15 (2)
Panic disorder	4 (5)	8 (5)	11 (4)	5 (2)	5 (3)	12(6)	2 (2)	24 (9)	8 (3)	11 (5)	9 (1)
Any neurotic disorder	186 (25)	210 (20)	185 (15)	212 (16)	204(18)	210(20)	201 (17)	227 (22)	152 (17)	144(16)	195 (7)
Rate per thousand in past twelve months (SE)											
Functional psychoses	-	5 (3)	7 (3)	11 (4)	4 (2)	3(2)	1 (1)	5 (3)	3 (2)	2 (2)	4 (1)
Alcohol dependence	68 (17)	45 (11)	28 (7)	16 (5)	24 (7)	4(2)	7 (3)	14 (5)	1 (1)	1 (1)	21 (2)
Drug dependence	56 (14)	29 (7)	19 (6)	14 (5)	13 (5)	3(2)	5 (3)	-	9 (4)	7 (5)	15 (2)
Men *Rate per thousand in past week(SE)*											
Mixed anxiety and depressive disorder	33 (12)	53 (11)	57 (10)	76 (12)	73(12)	45(10)	42 (10)	35 (8)	59 (14)	61(14)	54 (4)
GAD	6 (4)	15 (7)	25 (6)	28 (7)	33 (9)	49(11)	30 (9)	29 (10)	34 (10)	27 (9)	28 (2)
Depressive episode	8 (6)	23 (9)	13 (6)	10 (4)	15 (5)	18(6)	23 (7)	23 (8)	20 (7)	21 (7)	17 (2)
All phobias	4 (4)	11 (6)	9 (4)	5 (2)	5 (3)	3(2)	9 (4)	13 (5)	5 (2)	3 (2)	7 (1)
OCD	3 (3)	13 (6)	9 (4)	8 (3)	12 (4)	10(4)	11 (6)	11 (5)	8 (4)	5 (4)	9 (2)
Panic disorder	14 (8)	6 (4)	9 (6)	5 (3)	5 (3)	8(4)	9 (5)	14 (7)	3 (2)	5 (3)	8 (2)
Any neurotic disorder	68 (17)	122 (16)	122 (15)	133 (16)	143(15)	132(17)	125 (17)	125 (18)	129 (18)	122(17)	123 (5)
Rate per thousand in past twelve months (SE)											
Functional psychoses	3 (3)	5 (4)	5 (3)	3 (2)	4 (2)	2(2)	4 (3)	-	10 (6)	9 (6)	4 (1)
Alcohol dependence	113(23)	176 (22)	115 (16)	85 (13)	57(10)	53(11)	35 (9)	42 (11)	8 (4)	12 (5)	75 (5)
Drug dependence	79 (17)	111 (18)	26 (6)	28 (5)	13 (5)	16(6)	2 (1)	5 (3)	2 (2)	4 (4)	29 (3)
All adults *Rate per thousand in past week(SE)*											
Mixed anxiety and depressive disorder	60 (12)	82 (9)	81 (7)	100 (10)	94 (9)	79 (9)	76 (8)	63 (8)	54 (9)	58 (9)	77 (3)
GAD	5 (3)	19 (5)	24 (4)	27 (5)	32 (6)	42 (7)	34 (6)	45 (8)	41 (7)	46 (8)	31 (2)
Depressive episode	20 (7)	24 (6)	18 (4)	22 (4)	19 (4)	22 (5)	27 (5)	23 (5)	19 (5)	13 (3)	21 (1)
All phobias	24 (7)	12 (4)	10 (3)	10 (3)	12 (3)	6 (3)	11 (3)	12 (3)	8 (2)	4 (1)	11 (1)
OCD	8 (4)	21 (4)	11 (3)	9 (3)	13 (3)	13 (4)	10 (3)	15 (4)	14 (4)	4 (2)	12 (1)
Panic disorder	9 (5)	7 (3)	10 (4)	5 (2)	5 (2)	10 (3)	5 (3)	19 (6)	5 (2)	8 (3)	8 (1)
Any neurotic disorder	126 (15)	166 (13)	154 (10)	173 (12)	174(12)	172(14)	164 (14)	176 (14)	141 (13)	133(13)	160 (5)
Rate per thousand in past twelve months (SE)											
Functional psychoses	2 (2)	5 (3)	6 (2)	7 (2)	4 (2)	2(1)	2 (1)	3 (2)	6 (3)	5 (3)	4 (1)
Alcohol dependence	99 (15)	110 (12)	72 (9)	50 (7)	40 (7)	27(6)	21 (5)	28 (6)	4 (2)	7 (3)	47 (3)
Drug dependence	68 (11)	70 (10)	23 (4)	26 (4)	13 (3)	9(3)	4 (2)	2 (2)	5 (2)	4 (3)	22 (2)

GAD Generalised Anxiety Disorder;   OCD Obsessive-Compulsive Disorder

Table 6.2 Prevalence of psychiatric disorders by ethnicity and sex (rate per thousand population)

	Ethnicity*			All
	White	West Indian or African	Asian or Oriental	
	Rate per thousand in past week (SE)			
Women				
Mixed anxiety and depressive disorder	96 (5)	136 (34)	160 (45)	99 (5)
Generalised Anxiety Disorder	35 (3)	22 (16)	8 (8)	34 (3)
Depressive episode	24 (2)	6 (6)	51 (24)	25 (2)
All phobias	14 (2)	18 (15)	29 (10)	14 (2)
Obsessive-Compulsive Disorder	15 (2)	-	3 (3)	15 (2)
Panic disorder	9 (2)	7 (7)	7 (7)	9 (1)
Any neurotic disorder	194 (7)	190 (34)	258 (51)	195 (7)
	Rate per thousand in past twelve months (SE)			
Functional psychoses	4 (1)	34 (24)	-	4 (1)
Alcohol dependence	21 (2)	38 (24)	4 (4)	21 (2)
Drug dependence	15 (2)	33 (19)	-	15 (2)
	Rate per thousand in past week (SE)			
Men				
Mixed anxiety and depressive disorder	54 (4)	58 (28)	68 (27)	54 (4)
Generalised Anxiety Disorder	28 (2)	62 (39)	10 (10)	28 (2)
Depressive episode	17 (2)	21 (16)	19 (11)	17 (2)
All phobias	7 (1)	7 (8)	18 (13)	7 (1)
Obsessive-Compulsive Disorder	10 (2)	-	-	9 (2)
Panic disorder	8 (2)	7 (7)	-	8 (2)
Any neurotic disorder	124 (5)	155 (44)	115 (33)	123 (5)
	Rate per thousand in past twelve months (SE)			
Functional psychoses	4 (1)	7 (7)	2 (2)	4 (1)
Alcohol dependence	78 (5)	23 (17)	3 (4)	75 (5)
Drug dependence	28 (3)	68 (36)	36 (22)	29 (3)
	Rate per thousand in past week (SE)			
All adults				
Mixed anxiety and depressive disorder	75 (3)	99 (21)	112 (27)	77 (3)
Generalised Anxiety Disorder	31 (2)	41 (20)	9 (9)	31 (2)
Depressive episode	21 (2)	13 (8)	34 (13)	21 (1)
All phobias	10 (1)	13 (9)	23 (10)	11 (1)
Obsessive-Compulsive Disorder	13 (1)	-	2 (2)	12 (1)
Panic disorder	9 (1)	7 (5)	3 (3)	8 (1)
Any neurotic disorder	159 (5)	173 (27)	182 (32)	160 (5)
	Rate per thousand in past twelve months (SE)			
Functional psychoses	4 (1)	21 (13)	1 (1)	4 (1)
Alcohol dependence	49 (3)	31 (2)	4 (3)	47 (3)
Drug dependence	21 (2)	50 (19)	19 (13)	22 (2)

* Respondents who could not be classified into the three ethnic groups or refused to answer are included in the "All" category.

Table 6.3 Prevalence of psychiatric disorders by marital status and sex (rate per thousand population)

	Marital status*						All
	Married	Cohabiting	Single	Widowed	Divorced	Separated	
Rate per thousand in past week (SE)							
Women							
Mixed anxiety and depressive disorder	86 (6)	133 (19)	102 (10)	97 (23)	161 (17)	121 (21)	99 (5)
Generalised Anxiety Disorder	36 (4)	39 (11)	18 (4)	75 (19)	41 (10)	32 (12)	34 (3)
Depressive episode	17 (2)	30 (9)	33 (6)	38 (12)	46 (8)	56 (15)	25 (2)
All phobias	10 (2)	24 (8)	23 (5)	8 (5)	13 (5)	23 (11)	14 (2)
Obsessive-Compulsive Disorder	12 (2)	11 (6)	18 (5)	12 (6)	30 (9)	23 (9)	15 (2)
Panic disorder	8 (2)	3 (4)	7 (3)	38 (14)	13 (6)	8 (6)	9 (1)
Any neurotic disorder	170 (8)	240 (23)	201 (14)	268 (29)	304 (24)	263 (30)	195 (7)
Rate per thousand in past twelve months (SE)							
Functional psychoses	3 (1)	6 (4)	4 (2)	9 (5)	15 (6)	7 (6)	4 (1)
Alcohol dependence	9 (2)	28 (9)	51 (8)	15 (7)	23 (6)	26 (1)	21 (2)
Drug dependence	8 (2)	25 (9)	33 (6)	15 (7)	14 (5)	12 (7)	15 (2)
Rate per thousand in past week (SE)							
Men							
Mixed anxiety and depressive disorder	51 (5)	64 (15)	54 (6)	95 (39)	62 (14)	117 (34)	54 (4)
Generalised Anxiety Disorder	29 (3)	15 (7)	27 (5)	12 (12)	35 (12)	27 (15)	28 (2)
Depressive episode	14 (2)	11 (7)	16 (4)	70 (33)	37 (11)	111 (29)	17 (2)
All phobias	5 (1)	14 (7)	6 (2)	-	23 (8)	36 (19)	7 (1)
Obsessive-Compulsive Disorder	9 (2)	8 (6)	10 (3)	-	13 (6)	19 (20)	9 (2)
Panic disorder	7 (2)	4 (3)	10 (4)	24 (24)	8 (5)	-	8 (2)
Any neurotic disorder	116 (6)	115 (19)	123 (9)	200 (54)	178 (24)	309 (55)	123 (5)
Rate per thousand in past twelve months (SE)							
Functional psychoses	3 (1)	6 (5)	7 (2)	23 (17)	3 (3)	-	4 (1)
Alcohol dependence	39 (4)	89 (17)	144 (13)	65 (34)	95 (20)	200 (47)	75 (5)
Drug dependence	5 (2)	25 (9)	79 (9)	48 (30)	29 (13)	67 (34)	29 (3)
Rate per thousand in past week (SE)							
All adults							
Mixed anxiety and depressive disorder	69 (4)	100 (12)	74 (6)	96 (19)	123 (12)	120 (16)	77 (3)
Generalised Anxiety Disorder	32 (3)	28 (6)	23 (3)	63 (15)	39 (7)	31 (10)	31 (2)
Depressive episode	16 (2)	21 (6)	23 (4)	44 (11)	42 (6)	73 (15)	21 (1)
All phobias	8 (1)	19 (5)	13 (3)	6 (4)	17 (4)	27 (10)	11 (1)
Obsessive-Compulsive Disorder	10 (1)	9 (4)	13 (2)	10 (5)	23 (6)	21 (9)	12 (1)
Panic disorder	8 (1)	4 (2)	9 (3)	35 (13)	11 (4)	6 (4)	8 (1)
Any neurotic disorder	143 (6)	181 (15)	157 (8)	254 (26)	256 (16)	277 (27)	160 (5)
Rate per thousand in past twelve months (SE)							
Functional psychoses	3 (1)	6 (3)	5 (2)	11 (5)	10 (4)	5 (4)	4 (1)
Alcohol dependence	24 (2)	57 (9)	104 (8)	24 (9)	51 (9)	77 (2)	47 (3)
Drug dependence	6 (2)	25 (1)	59 (6)	22 (1)	20 (1)	29 (1)	22 (2)

* Respondents with insufficient information to code marital status are included in the "All" category.

Table 6.4 Prevalence of psychiatric disorders by age when finished full time education and sex (rate per thousand population)

	Age when finished full time education*							All
	Not yet finished	14 or under	15	16	17	18	19 or over	
	Rate per thousand in past week (SE)							
Women								
Mixed anxiety and depressive disorder	92 (26)	92 (16)	101 (10)	104 (9)	88 (14)	80 (13)	107 (12)	99 (5)
Generalised Anxiety Disorder	-	77 (15)	54 (6)	23 (4)	26 (8)	31 (8)	23 (6)	34 (3)
Depressive episode	42 (19)	24 (9)	30 (5)	25 (4)	21 (6)	9 (4)	21 (4)	25 (2)
All phobias	66 (19)	11 (5)	18 (4)	9 (2)	12 (5)	14 (6)	7 (3)	14 (2)
Obsessive-Compulsive Disorder	14 (10)	12 (6)	18 (4)	15 (3)	17 (6)	10 (5)	12 (4)	15 (2)
Panic disorder	7 (7)	19 (8)	11 (3)	7 (2)	8 (4)	6 (3)	8 (4)	9 (1)
Any neurotic disorder	221 (34)	236 (22)	231 (14)	184 (11)	172 (21)	149 (17)	177 (14)	195 (7)
	Rate per thousand in past twelve months (SE)							
Functional psychoses	-	4 (3)	3 (2)	5 (2)	5 (3)	8 (4)	4 (2)	4 (1)
Alcohol dependence	82 (24)	7 (6)	16 (4)	21 (4)	16 (6)	14 (6)	20 (6)	21 (2)
Drug dependence	50 (15)	20 (8)	10 (3)	12 (3)	15 (6)	13 (5)	16 (6)	15 (2)
	Rate per thousand in past week (SE)							
Men								
Mixed anxiety and depressive disorder	55 (16)	55 (11)	52 (7)	58 (7)	36 (10)	53 (14)	60 (9)	54 (4)
Generalised Anxiety Disorder	8 (8)	42 (12)	36 (7)	24 (4)	18 (8)	30 (11)	23 (5)	28 (2)
Depressive episode	24 (12)	32 (8)	28 (6)	12 (3)	10 (6)	3 (2)	11 (4)	17 (2)
All phobias	10 (7)	6 (3)	10 (3)	9 (3)	-	3 (3)	4 (2)	7 (1)
Obsessive-Compulsive Disorder	6 (6)	10 (6)	13 (3)	9 (2)	6 (4)	6 (4)	10 (4)	9 (2)
Panic disorder	6 (6)	8 (6)	12 (4)	2 (2)	5 (4)	12 (9)	12 (4)	8 (2)
Any neurotic disorder	109 (22)	153 (18)	150 (12)	115 (9)	75 (14)	108 (19)	120 (12)	123 (5)
	Rate per thousand in past twelve months (SE)							
Functional psychoses	4 (4)	12 (8)	-	4 (2)	-	11 (8)	4 (2)	4 (1)
Alcohol dependence	78 (22)	26 (8)	66 (8)	101 (8)	70 (16)	59 (15)	67 (11)	75 (5)
Drug dependence	80 (22)	13 (6)	27 (6)	33 (5)	22 (9)	21 (10)	20 (6)	29 (3)
	Rate per thousand in past week (SE)							
All adults								
Mixed anxiety and depressive disorder	72 (16)	74 (9)	77 (6)	81 (6)	65 (9)	68 (11)	82 (8)	77 (3)
Generalised Anxiety Disorder	4 (4)	60 (10)	45 (5)	24 (3)	23 (6)	31 (6)	23 (4)	31 (2)
Depressive episode	32 (11)	28 (6)	29 (4)	18 (2)	16 (4)	6 (2)	16 (3)	21 (1)
All phobias	37 (10)	8 (2)	14 (2)	9 (2)	7 (3)	9 (4)	6 (2)	11 (1)
Obsessive-Compulsive Disorder	10 (6)	11 (4)	15 (3)	12 (2)	12 (4)	8 (3)	11 (3)	12 (1)
Panic disorder	6 (4)	14 (5)	11 (2)	5 (1)	6 (3)	9 (4)	10 (3)	8 (1)
Any neurotic disorder	161 (20)	194 (15)	191 (9)	149 (7)	130 (14)	132 (15)	147 (10)	160 (5)
	Rate per thousand in past twelve months (SE)							
Functional psychoses	2 (2)	8 (4)	2 (1)	5 (1)	3 (2)	9 (4)	4 (2)	4 (1)
Alcohol dependence	80 (16)	17 (5)	41 (5)	62 (5)	39 (8)	32 (7)	45 (7)	47 (3)
Drug dependence	66 (13)	17 (5)	18 (3)	23 (3)	18 (5)	16 (5)	18 (4)	22 (2)

* No answers and those who had never been to school are excluded from the seven age categories but included in the "All" category.

Table 6.5 Prevalence of psychiatric disorders by educational qualifications and sex (rate per thousand population)

	Educational qualifications*						All
	Degree	Teaching/ HND/ Nursing	A Level	GCSE, grades A-C or equivalent	GCSE, grades D-F or equivalent	No qualifications	
Rate per thousand in past week (SE)							
Women							
Mixed anxiety and depressive disorder	83 (13)	107 (18)	119 (15)	93 (8)	115 (15)	94 (8)	99 (5)
Generalised Anxiety Disorder	28 (8)	29 (8)	17 (7)	28 (5)	21 (5)	51 (5)	34 (3)
Depressive episode	25 (6)	14 (4)	27 (10)	19 (4)	23 (5)	33 (4)	25 (2)
All phobias	8 (4)	10 (5)	11 (5)	17 (5)	11 (4)	18 (3)	14 (2)
Obsessive-Compulsive Disorder	11 (4)	5 (3)	12 (7)	15 (4)	18 (6)	17 (3)	15 (2)
Panic disorder	9 (6)	4 (3)	8 (4)	8 (3)	7 (4)	12 (3)	9 (1)
Any neurotic disorder	164 (19)	169 (20)	194 (18)	180 (11)	195 (19)	224 (11)	195 (7)
Rate per thousand in past twelve months (SE)							
Functional psychoses	5 (3)	3 (2)	8 (4)	5 (2)	5 (2)	3 (1)	4 (1)
Alcohol dependence	28 (8)	16 (8)	31 (11)	20 (4)	20 (6)	17 (3)	21 (2)
Drug dependence	8 (4)	12 (5)	23 (7)	17 (4)	16 (5)	14 (3)	15 (2)
Rate per thousand in past week (SE)							
Men							
Mixed anxiety and depressive disorder	51 (9)	45 (8)	74 (12)	61 (8)	35 (8)	52 (7)	54 (4)
Generalised Anxiety Disorder	33 (7)	19 (5)	26 (8)	20 (4)	37 (10)	35 (6)	28 (2)
Depressive episode	5 (2)	15 (6)	7 (3)	19 (5)	22 (8)	25 (5)	17 (2)
All phobias	5 (2)	2 (2)	7 (4)	7 (2)	10 (5)	10 (2)	7 (1)
Obsessive-Compulsive Disorder	14 (5)	5 (3)	6 (4)	8 (2)	6 (3)	14 (4)	9 (2)
Panic disorder	12 (5)	5 (3)	9 (7)	4 (2)	6 (4)	10 (3)	8 (2)
Any neurotic disorder	120 (13)	91 (12)	130 (16)	120 (11)	116 (17)	145 (11)	123 (5)
Rate per thousand in past twelve months (SE)							
Functional psychoses	2 (2)	1 (1)	10 (4)	5 (3)	3 (2)	4 (2)	4 (1)
Alcohol dependence	56 (12)	76 (12)	88 (12)	95 (10)	90 (14)	53 (8)	75 (5)
Drug dependence	7 (3)	21 (7)	44 (10)	42 (8)	34 (10)	22 (5)	29 (3)
Rate per thousand in past week (SE)							
All adults							
Mixed anxiety and depressive disorder	64 (8)	70 (9)	93 (10)	78 (6)	79 (9)	76 (6)	77 (3)
Generalised Anxiety Disorder	31 (5)	23 (5)	22 (5)	24 (3)	28 (6)	44 (4)	31 (2)
Depressive episode	13 (3)	15 (4)	16 (4)	19 (3)	23 (4)	29 (3)	21 (1)
All phobias	6 (2)	5 (2)	8 (3)	13 (3)	10 (4)	14 (2)	11 (1)
Obsessive-Compulsive disorder	13 (4)	5 (2)	9 (4)	12 (2)	12 (4)	15 (2)	12 (1)
Panic disorder	11 (4)	5 (2)	9 (4)	6 (2)	7 (2)	11 (2)	8 (1)
Any neurotic disorder	138 (12)	122 (12)	157 (12)	152 (8)	160 (14)	190 (9)	160 (5)
Rate per thousand in past twelve months (SE)							
Functional psychoses	3 (2)	2 (1)	9 (3)	5 (2)	4 (2)	3 (1)	4 (1)
Alcohol dependence	44 (9)	52 (8)	64 (8)	55 (6)	52 (7)	33 (4)	47 (3)
Drug dependence	8 (3)	18 (5)	35 (7)	29 (4)	24 (6)	17 (3)	22 (2)

* For details of educational qualifications see Glossary

Table 6.6 Prevalence of psychiatric disorders by employment status and sex (rate per thousand population)

	Employment status				All	
	Working full-time	Working part-time	Unemployed	Economically inactive		
Rate per thousand in past week (SE)						
Women						
Mixed anxiety and depressive disorder	94 (8)	88 (8)	206 (27)	94 (8)	99 (5)	
Generalised Anxiety Disorder	29 (4)	27 (5)	60 (15)	41 (4)	34 (3)	
Depressive episode	11 (2)	22 (4)	56 (13)	37 (5)	25 (2)	
All phobias	8 (2)	12 (3)	23 (10)	22 (4)	14 (2)	
Obsessive-Compulsive Disorder	13 (3)	13 (3)	27 (10)	16 (3)	15 (2)	
Panic disorder	9 (3)	7 (3)	9 (4)	10 (2)	9 (1)	
Any neurotic disorder	164 (11)	168 (11)	381 (34)	220 (11)	195 (7)	
Rate per thousand in past twelve months (SE)						
Functional psychoses	2 (1)	4 (2)	10 (5)	7 (2)	5 (1)	
Alcohol dependence	18 (3)	31 (6)	28 (14)	18 (4)	22 (2)	
Drug dependence	7 (2)	11 (3)	55 (14)	20 (4)	15 (2)	
Rate per thousand in past week (SE)						
Men						
Mixed anxiety and depressive disorder	46 (4)	56 (16)	80 (12)	76 (11)	54 (4)	
Generalised Anxiety Disorder	21 (3)	29 (17)	51 (10)	37 (7)	28 (2)	
Depressive episode	12 (2)	16 (10)	27 (8)	37 (8)	17 (2)	
All phobias	4 (1)	5 (4)	17 (6)	14 (4)	7 (1)	
Obsessive-Compulsive Disorder	7 (1)	6 (5)	16 (5)	20 (6)	9 (2)	
Panic disorder	6 (2)	5 (5)	12 (6)	12 (4)	8 (2)	
Any neurotic disorder	95 (6)	117 (25)	203 (18)	195 (18)	123 (5)	
Rate per thousand in past twelve months (SE)						
Functional psychoses	2 (1)	10 (8)	6 (3)	14 (5)	4 (1)	
Alcohol dependence	74 (6)	91 (21)	117 (16)	56 (10)	77 (5)	
Drug dependence	15 (3)	51 (17)	96 (16)	29 (6)	29 (3)	
Rate per thousand in past week (SE)						
All adults						
Mixed anxiety and depressive disorder	62 (4)	83 (7)	120 (13)	89 (7)	77 (3)	
Generalised Anxiety Disorder	24 (3)	27 (5)	54 (9)	40 (4)	31 (2)	
Depressive episode	11 (1)	21 (4)	36 (6)	37 (4)	21 (1)	
All phobias	5 (1)	11 (3)	19 (5)	20 (3)	11 (1)	
Obsessive-Compulsive Disorder	9 (1)	12 (3)	19 (5)	17 (3)	12 (1)	
Panic disorder	7 (1)	7 (2)	11 (4)	11 (2)	8 (1)	
Any neurotic disorder	118 (6)	160 (10)	259 (17)	212 (10)	160 (5)	
Rate per thousand in past twelve months (SE)						
Functional psychoses	2 (1)	5 (2)	7 (2)	9 (2)	4 (1)	
Alcohol dependence	54 (4)	42 (6)	89 (13)	29 (4)	49 (3)	
Drug dependence	13 (2)	17 (4)	83 (12)	23 (3)	22 (2)	

Table 6.7 Prevalence of psychiatric disorders by social class (based on occupation of head of family unit) and sex (rate per thousand population)

	Social class*						All§
	I	II	III NM	III M	IV	V	
	Rate per thousand in past week (SE)						
Women							
Mixed anxiety and depressive disorder	98 (19)	91 (9)	101 (11)	101 (10)	109 (12)	98 (20)	99 (5)
Generalised Anxiety Disorder	23 (10)	27 (5)	39 (7)	34 (4)	44 (8)	52 (18)	34 (3)
Depressive episode	16 (7)	12 (2)	32 (6)	26 (4)	39 (8)	24 (10)	25 (2)
All phobias	-	8 (2)	17 (4)	11 (3)	24 (6)	20 (10)	14 (2)
Obsessive-Compulsive Disorder	15 (8)	10 (3)	12 (4)	15 (4)	12 (4)	43 (15)	15 (2)
Panic disorder	3 (3)	8 (3)	12 (3)	11 (3)	6 (3)	10 (5)	9 (1)
Any neurotic disorder	155 (21)	154 (11)	213 (15)	198 (12)	235 (17)	247 (31)	195 (7)
	Rate per thousand in past twelve months (SE)						
Functional psychoses	7 (5)	3 (1)	1 (1)	6 (2)	4 (2)	16 (8)	4 (1)
Alcohol dependence	17 (8)	11 (3)	32 (7)	14 (4)	28 (6)	32 (13)	21 (2)
Drug dependence	11 (7)	7 (2)	25 (6)	10 (3)	20 (5)	26 (10)	14 (2)
	Rate per thousand in past week (SE)						
Men							
Mixed anxiety and depressive disorder	31 (9)	60 (8)	66 (12)	58 (7)	40 (7)	51 (14)	54 (4)
Generalised Anxiety Disorder	22 (8)	29 (4)	30 (7)	26 (5)	37 (9)	13 (9)	28 (2)
Depressive episode	4 (3)	12 (3)	24 (8)	18 (3)	16 (5)	44 (16)	17 (2)
All phobias	3 (2)	8 (2)	8 (3)	5 (2)	13 (4)	7 (5)	7 (1)
Obsessive-Compulsive Disorder	-	15 (4)	7 (3)	10 (3)	10 (4)	-	9 (2)
Panic disorder	-	10 (3)	4 (3)	7 (3)	8 (4)	14 (8)	8 (2)
Any neurotic disorder	60 (14)	135 (10)	139 (15)	124 (9)	124 (13)	129 (27)	123 (5)
	Rate per thousand in past twelve months (SE)						
Functional psychoses	1 (2)	2 (1)	7 (5)	3 (1)	5 (3)	17 (9)	4 (1)
Alcohol dependence	45 (11)	60 (8)	76 (14)	74 (7)	92 (13)	110 (28)	73 (5)
Drug dependence	5 (4)	14 (4)	29 (8)	24 (5)	51 (10)	73 (20)	27 (3)
	Rate per thousand in past week (SE)						
All adults							
Mixed anxiety and depressive disorder	60 (10)	76 (6)	87 (7)	78 (6)	76 (7)	73 (11)	77 (3)
Generalised Anxiety Disorder	23 (6)	28 (3)	35 (5)	30 (3)	41 (6)	31 (10)	31 (2)
Depressive episode	9 (4)	12 (2)	29 (5)	22 (3)	28 (5)	35 (9)	21 (1)
All phobias	2 (1)	8 (2)	13 (3)	8 (2)	19 (4)	13 (5)	11 (1)
Obsessive-Compulsive Disorder	6 (3)	13 (2)	10 (3)	12 (2)	11 (2)	21 (7)	12 (1)
Panicdisorder	1 (2)	9 (2)	9 (2)	8 (2)	7 (2)	12 (5)	8 (1)
Any neurotic disorder	102 (12)	145 (8)	182 (11)	158 (8)	182 (12)	185 (18)	160 (5)
	Rate per thousand in past twelve months (SE)						
Functional psychoses	4 (2)	3 (1)	4 (2)	4 (1)	4 (1)	17 (6)	4 (1)
Alcohol dependence	33 (7)	34 (4)	50 (7)	47 (5)	58 (7)	73 (15)	46 (3)
Drug dependence	7 (4)	11 (2)	27 (5)	17 (3)	35 (5)	50 (11)	21 (2)

* I = Professional; II = Employers and Managers; IIINM = Intermediate and Junior non-manual. IIIM = Skilled manual and own account non-professional; IV = Semi-skilled Manual and Personal service; V = Unskilled manual.

§ No answers, Members of the Armed Forces, full-time students and those who have never worked are excluded from the six social class categories but included in the "All" category.

Table 6.8 Prevalence of psychiatric disorders by family unit type and sex (rate per thousand population)

	Family unit type*						All	
	Couple, no child	Couple & child(ren)	Lone parent & child(ren)	One person only	Adult with parents	Adult with one parent		
Women	*Rate per thousand in past week (SE)*							
Mixed anxiety and depressive disorder	75 (7)	102 (8)	146 (14)	143 (13)	60 (15)	73 (31)	99 (5)	
Generalised Anxiety Disorder	37 (5)	35 (4)	34 (8)	37 (6)	14 (8)	28 (16)	34 (3)	
Depressive episode	12 (3)	23 (3)	51 (8)	38 (6)	14 (8)	62 (30)	25 (2)	
All phobias	13 (3)	11 (2)	18 (4)	11 (3)	39 (12)	-	14 (2)	
Obsessive-Compulsive Disorder	15 (3)	10 (2)	20 (6)	23 (6)	13 (8)	34 (19)	15 (2)	
Panic disorder	5 (2)	9 (2)	20 (6)	8 (3)	10 (7)	-	9 (1)	
Any neurotic disorder	157 (11)	190 (10)	288 (17)	250 (18)	150 (22)	197 (44)	195 (7)	
	Rate per thousand in past twelve months (SE)							
Functional psychoses	-	6 (2)	12 (4)	10 (3)	-	-	4 (1)	
Alcohol dependence	9 (3)	13 (3)	28 (7)	49 (8)	30 (11)	77 (32)	21 (2)	
Drug dependence	8 (3)	10 (3)	26 (7)	27 (6)	24 (9)	39 (21)	15 (2)	
Men	*Rate per thousand in past week (SE)*							
Mixed anxiety and depressive disorder	48 (6)	55 (6)	83 (32)	75 (9)	34 (9)	72 (24)	54 (4)	
Generalised Anxiety Disorder	20 (4)	33 (4)	36 (23)	38 (7)	15 (8)	28 (11)	28 (2)	
Depressive episode	14 (4)	14 (3)	33 (15)	28 (6)	22 (8)	8 (6)	17 (2)	
All phobias	8 (2)	5 (2)	17 (17)	12 (3)	3 (4)	13 (9)	7 (1)	
Obsessive-Compulsive Disorder	8 (2)	9 (2)	17 (18)	17 (4)	5 (4)	8 (6)	9 (2)	
Panic disorder	9 (3)	5 (2)	33 (24)	6 (3)	8 (5)	20 (15)	8 (2)	
Any neurotic disorder	109 (10)	120 (8)	219 (53)	175 (12)	87 (14)	149 (28)	123 (5)	
	Rate per thousand in past twelve months (SE)							
Functional psychoses	4 (2)	2 (2)	-	12 (3)	3 (4)	5 (2)	4 (1)	
Alcohol dependence	47 (7)	41 (6)	129 (42)	145 (13)	128 (21)	142 (28)	75 (5)	
Drug dependence	5 (3)	8 (2)	10 (10)	72 (11)	74 (15)	81 (19)	29 (3)	
All adults	*Rate per thousand in past week (SE)*							
Mixed anxiety and depressive disorder	63 (5)	78 (5)	139 (13)	101 (7)	44 (8)	72 (19)	77 (3)	
Generalised Anxiety Disorder	29 (3)	34 (3)	34 (7)	37 (5)	14 (6)	28 (9)	31 (2)	
Depressive episode	13 (2)	18 (2)	49 (8)	32 (4)	19 (6)	27 (12)	21 (1)	
All phobias	11 (2)	8 (2)	17 (4)	12 (2)	17 (5)	8 (6)	11 (1)	
Obsessive-Compulsive Disorder	12 (2)	9 (2)	19 (6)	19 (3)	8 (4)	17 (8)	12 (1)	
Panic disorder	7 (2)	7 (2)	21 (6)	7 (2)	9 (4)	13 (10)	8 (1)	
Any neurotic disorder	134 (8)	155 (7)	281 (16)	209 (10)	112 (12)	166 (24)	160 (5)	
	Rate per thousand in past twelve months (SE)							
Functional psychoses	2 (1)	4 (1)	11 (3)	11 (2)	2 (2)	3 (1)	4 (1)	
Alcohol dependence	27 (4)	27 (3)	38 (8)	102 (8)	89 (14)	118 (20)	47 (3)	
Drug dependence	7 (2)	9 (2)	24 (6)	52 (7)	55 (10)	66 (15)	22 (2)	

* For details of family unit type, see Glossary.

Table 6.9 Prevalence of psychiatric disorders by tenure and sex (rate per thousand population)

	Tenure				All
	Owned outright	Owned with mortgage	Rented from HA or LA	Rented from other source	
	Rate per thousand in past week (SE)				
Women					
Mixed anxiety and depressive disorder	62 (8)	92 (7)	140 (12)	115 (15)	99 (5)
Generalised Anxiety Disorder	39 (8)	27 (3)	49 (7)	29 (8)	34 (3)
Depressive episode	21 (5)	20 (3)	37 (6)	33 (9)	25 (2)
All phobias	9 (3)	15 (3)	18 (4)	12 (4)	14 (2)
Obsessive-Compulsive Disorder	8 (3)	15 (2)	19 (4)	18 (8)	15 (2)
Panic disorder	9 (4)	7 (2)	15 (3)	4 (3)	9 (1)
Any neurotic disorder	148 (14)	176 (8)	278 (16)	212 (20)	195 (7)
	Rate per thousand in past twelve months (SE)				
Functional psychoses	2 (1)	2 (1)	10 (3)	11 (17)	4 (1)
Alcohol dependence	19 (6)	14 (3)	28 (6)	46 (18)	21 (2)
Drug dependence	6 (3)	11 (2)	31 (6)	24 (19)	15 (2)
	Rate per thousand in past week (SE)				
Men					
Mixed anxiety and depressive disorder	41 (8)	49 (5)	75 (10)	71 (12)	54 (4)
Generalised Anxiety Disorder	23 (6)	23 (3)	40 (8)	43 (10)	28 (2)
Depressive episode	11 (4)	12 (2)	40 (8)	18 (7)	17 (2)
All phobias	4 (2)	6 (2)	16 (5)	4 (2)	7 (1)
Obsessive-Compulsive Disorder	14 (6)	7 (2)	12 (3)	11 (4)	9 (2)
Panic disorder	6 (3)	4 (1)	18 (6)	12 (6)	8 (2)
Any neurotic disorder	99 (11)	102 (7)	202 (14)	158 (17)	123 (5)
	Rate per thousand in past twelve months (SE)				
Functional psychoses	2 (2)	3 (1)	9 (4)	6 (14)	4 (1)
Alcohol dependence	38 (8)	68 (6)	100 (16)	132 (24)	75 (5)
Drug dependence	19 (5)	17 (3)	54 (11)	70 (12)	29 (3)
	Rate per thousand in past week (SE)				
All adults					
Mixed anxiety and depressive disorder	52 (6)	70 (4)	111 (7)	92 (10)	77 (3)
Generalised Anxiety Disorder	31 (5)	25 (2)	45 (6)	36 (6)	31 (2)
Depressive episode	17 (3)	16 (2)	39 (4)	25 (6)	21 (1)
All phobias	7 (2)	10 (2)	17 (4)	8 (2)	11 (1)
Obsessive-Compulsive Disorder	11 (3)	11 (1)	16 (3)	14 (4)	12 (1)
Panic disorder	8 (3)	6 (1)	16 (3)	8 (4)	8 (1)
Any neurotic disorder	125 (10)	138 (6)	244 (11)	184 (13)	160 (5)
	Rate per thousand in past twelve months (SE)				
Functional psychoses	2 (1)	3 (1)	10 (2)	8 (11)	4 (1)
Alcohol dependence	28 (5)	42 (3)	60 (8)	92 (14)	47 (3)
Drug dependence	12 (3)	14 (2)	42 (6)	48 (12)	22 (2)

Table 6.10 Prevalence of psychiatric disorders by type of accommodation and sex (rate per thousand population)

	Type of accommodation				All	
	Detached	Semi-detached	Terraced	Flat or maisonette		
Rate per thousand in past week (SE)						
Women						
Mixed anxiety and depressive disorder	72 (10)	77 (7)	122 (9)	137 (12)	99 (5)	
Generalised Anxiety Disorder	26 (5)	34 (5)	35 (4)	44 (7)	34 (3)	
Depressive episode	18 (4)	21 (4)	28 (4)	36 (6)	25 (2)	
All phobias	13 (4)	12 (3)	17 (3)	16 (4)	14 (2)	
Obsessive-Compulsive Disorder	13 (3)	13 (3)	14 (3)	20 (5)	15 (2)	
Panic disorder	8 (3)	9 (2)	10 (2)	8 (3)	9 (1)	
Any neurotic disorder	149 (14)	166 (10)	225 (12)	260 (16)	195 (7)	
Rate per thousand in past twelve months (SE)						
Functional psychoses	4 (2)	4 (2)	4 (1)	8 (3)	4 (1)	
Alcohol dependence	12 (4)	9 (3)	29 (5)	41 (8)	21 (2)	
Drug dependence	5 (3)	11 (3)	13 (3)	42 (9)	15 (2)	
Rate per thousand in past week (SE)						
Men						
Mixed anxiety and depressive disorder	50 (8)	50 (6)	54 (7)	72 (8)	54 (4)	
Generalised Anxiety Disorder	24 (5)	28 (5)	28 (5)	34 (6)	28 (2)	
Depressive episode	8 (3)	15 (3)	21 (5)	28 (6)	17 (2)	
All phobias	3 (1)	4 (2)	9 (3)	15 (4)	7 (1)	
Obsessive-Compulsive Disorder	7 (2)	5 (2)	13 (4)	17 (4)	9 (2)	
Panic disorder	5 (3)	6 (2)	8 (3)	13 (4)	8 (2)	
Any neurotic disorder	97 (10)	109 (8)	133 (10)	179 (12)	123 (5)	
Rate per thousand in past twelve months (SE)						
Functional psychoses	1 (1)	7 (3)	2 (1)	8 (3)	4 (1)	
Alcohol dependence	43 (9)	63 (7)	95 (9)	108 (15)	75 (5)	
Drug dependence	14 (5)	20 (5)	45 (7)	37 (8)	29 (3)	
Rate per thousand in past week (SE)						
All adults						
Mixed anxiety and depressive disorder	61 (7)	63 (5)	89 (6)	106 (8)	77 (3)	
Generalised Anxiety Disorder	25 (4)	31 (4)	31 (3)	39 (5)	31 (2)	
Depressive episode	13 (2)	18 (2)	24 (3)	32 (4)	21 (1)	
All phobias	8 (2)	8 (2)	13 (2)	16 (3)	11 (1)	
Obsessive Compulsive Disorder	10 (2)	9 (2)	13 (2)	19 (4)	12 (1)	
Panic disorder	6 (2)	8 (2)	9 (2)	11 (3)	8 (1)	
Any neurotic disorder	123 (9)	137 (7)	180 (8)	221 (11)	160 (5)	
Rate per thousand in past twelve months (SE)						
Functional psychoses	2 (1)	5 (1)	3 (1)	8 (2)	4 (1)	
Alcohol dependence	27 (5)	37 (4)	61 (5)	73 (8)	47 (3)	
Alcohol dependence	10 (3)	16 (3)	29 (4)	39 (6)	22 (2)	

85

Table 6.11 Prevalence of psychiatric disorders by Regional Health Authority (RHA) and sex (rate per thousand population)

	RHA								
	Northern	Yorkshire	Trent	East Anglia	NW Thames	NE Thames	SE Thames	SW Thames	Wessex

Rate per thousand in past week (SE)

Women

	Northern	Yorkshire	Trent	East Anglia	NW Thames	NE Thames	SE Thames	SW Thames	Wessex
Mixed anxiety and depressive disorder	109 (20)	110 (21)	66 (12)	75 (21)	110 (22)	150 (23)	112 (20)	139 (24)	59 (15)
Generalised Anxiety Disorder	46 (9)	42 (11)	31 (6)	43 (16)	30 (10)	44 (13)	44 (13)	13 (8)	16 (9)
Depressive episode	24 (7)	33 (8)	14 (6)	36 (10)	23 (8)	35 (14)	28 (9)	20 (8)	13 (6)
All phobias	15 (14)	8 (6)	16 (5)	10 (6)	9 (4)	8 (5)	18 (8)	34 (11)	17 (10)
Obsessive-Compulsive Disorder	13 (8)	10 (5)	6 (3)	19 (9)	9 (6)	24 (8)	13 (6)	8 (9)	29 (8)
Panic disorder	4 (3)	13 (6)	1 (1)	8 (8)	14 (5)	13 (4)	6 (5)	2 (2)	12 (8)
Any neurotic disorder	210 (35)	216 (31)	134 (15)	190 (34)	196 (31)	275 (27)	221 (28)	215 (40)	145 (28)

Rate per thousand in past twelve months (SE)

	Northern	Yorkshire	Trent	East Anglia	NW Thames	NE Thames	SE Thames	SW Thames	Wessex
Functional psychoses	2 (1)	1 (2)	1 (1)	2 (2)	5 (4)	3 (2)	10 (5)	2 (6)	5 (4)
Alcohol dependence	22 (8)	25 (9)	11 (4)	17 (9)	13 (5)	34 (12)	26 (8)	11 (9)	16 (6)
Drug dependence	4 (3)	11 (6)	13 (7)	15 (15)	14 (9)	21 (1)	19 (7)	17 (7)	17 (7)

Rate per thousand in past week (SE)

Men

	Northern	Yorkshire	Trent	East Anglia	NW Thames	NE Thames	SE Thames	SW Thames	Wessex
Mixed anxiety and depressive disorder	63 (20)	20 (6)	65 (17)	47 (18)	44 (16)	48 (14)	62 (16)	53 (20)	62 (18)
Generalised Anxiety Disorder	38 (7)	39 (10)	31 (10)	15 (6)	29 (8)	30 (9)	31 (9)	42 (14)	3 (4)
Depressive episode	15 (6)	21 (8)	12 (6)	6 (6)	16 (6)	25 (8)	6 (5)	12 (6)	20 (12)
All phobias	2 (2)	2 (2)	9 (3)	-	9 (5)	6 (3)	7 (4)	15 (7)	6 (4)
Obsessive-Compulsive Disorder	9 (7)	14 (5)	7 (4)	-	14 (6)	5 (3)	19 (6)	4 (3)	11 (6)
Panic disorder	6 (5)	9 (7)	10 (5)	7 (7)	6 (4)	17 (12)	-	9 (8)	7 (7)
Any neurotic disorder	132 (28)	104 (12)	134 (19)	75 (25)	119 (19)	131 (18)	125 (18)	135 (20)	110 (25)

Rate per thousand in past twelve months (SE)

	Northern	Yorkshire	Trent	East Anglia	NW Thames	NE Thames	SE Thames	SW Thames	Wessex
Functional psychoses	4 (3)	5 (3)	2 (2)	6 (6)	4 (3)	-	8 (4)	2 (2)	-
Alcohol dependence	76 (26)	73 (23)	55 (15)	40 (10)	67 (12)	90 (17)	73 (13)	63 (21)	69 (15)
Drug dependence	13 (7)	17 (10)	26 (9)	10 (4)	30 (10)	54 (12)	36 (11)	27 (13)	27 (12)

Rate per thousand in past week (SE)

All adults

	Northern	Yorkshire	Trent	East Anglia	NW Thames	NE Thames	SE Thames	SW Thames	Wessex
Mixed anxiety and depressive disorder	86 (14)	67 (11)	65 (10)	62 (17)	77 (15)	97 (15)	88 (16)	95 (9)	61 (15)
Generalised anxiety disorder	42 (6)	41 (9)	31 (6)	30 (8)	30 (8)	37 (9)	38 (6)	28 (7)	10 (5)
Depressive episode	19 (4)	27 (6)	13 (4)	22 (7)	19 (4)	30 (6)	17 (6)	15 (7)	17 (6)
All phobias	8 (7)	5 (3)	12 (3)	5 (3)	9 (3)	7 (2)	12 (6)	24 (5)	11 (4)
Obsessive-Compulsive Disorder	11 (3)	12 (4)	6 (2)	10 (5)	11 (4)	14 (4)	16 (4)	6 (4)	20 (4)
Panic disorder	5 (3)	11 (5)	6 (3)	7 (8)	10 (3)	15 (6)	3 (3)	6 (4)	9 (6)
Any neurotic disorder	171 (26)	162 (18)	134 (12)	138 (29)	157 (19)	201 (20)	175 (18)	174 (16)	128 (22)

Rate per thousand in past twelve months (SE)

	Northern	Yorkshire	Trent	East Anglia	NW Thames	NE Thames	SE Thames	SW Thames	Wessex
Functional psycoses	3 (2)	3 (2)	2 (1)	4 (3)	4 (20)	2 (1)	9 (5)	7 (3)	3 (2)
Alcohol dependence	49 (15)	48 (12)	34 (9)	28 (4)	40 (7)	62 (13)	48 (10)	38 (13)	42 (9)
Drug dependence	8 (5)	14 (6)	20 (7)	12 (10)	22 (7)	38 (7)	27 (8)	22 (9)	22 (6)

Oxford	South Western	West Midlands	Mersey	North Western	England	Scotland	Wales	All	
									Women
									Mixed anxiety and
64 (17)	83 (13)	101 (19)	136 (27)	83 (16)	99 (5)	89 (22)	106 (19)	99 (5)	depressive disorder
									Generalised
33 (10)	21 (7)	28 (9)	51 (14)	33 (12)	34 (3)	23 (8)	54 (12)	34 (3)	Anxiety Disorder
7 (6)	28 (8)	34 (8)	38 (11)	24 (6)	25 (2)	25 (9)	15 (8)	25 (2)	Depressive episode
29 (10)	2 (2)	17 (7)	10 (6)	14 (7)	15 (2)	11 (5)	14 (8)	14 (2)	All phobias
									Obsessive-
4 (5)	12 (9)	16 (6)	21 (7)	11 (4)	14 (2)	14 (7)	30 (10)	15 (2)	Compulsive Disorder
9 (8)	5 (5)	10 (4)	4 (3)	20 (8)	9 (2)	15 (7)	-	9 (1)	Panic disorder
147 (30)	151 (12)	206 (25)	260 (39)	184 (22)	195 (8)	178 (27)	218 (31)	195 (7)	**Any neurotic disorder**
2 (2)	-	2 (2)	-	7 (6)	4 (1)	11 (6)	6 (4)	4 (1)	**Functional psychoses**
19 (12)	22 (7)	32 (8)	20 (11)	16 (10)	21 (2)	21 (8)	20 (13)	21 (2)	**Alcohol dependence**
13 (9)	12 (6)	19 (7)	9 (5)	18 (6)	15 (2)	16 (8)	22 (14)	15 (2)	**Drug dependence**
									Men
									Mixed anxiety and
57 (15)	64 (20)	82 (13)	47 (17)	48 (12)	56 (4)	55 (12)	32 (13)	54 (4)	depressive disorder
									Generalised
23 (7)	14 (7)	30 (11)	54 (14)	11 (7)	28 (3)	27 (11)	26 (12)	28 (2)	Anxiety Disorder
17 (11)	9 (7)	16 (7)	24 (5)	26 (13)	16 (2)	16 (5)	34 (13)	17 (2)	Depressive episode
11 (12)	8 (4)	2 (1)	11 (12)	11 (5)	7 (1)	9 (5)	5 (5)	7 (1)	All phobias
									Obsessive-
8 (5)	2 (2)	5 (3)	20 (10)	3 (2)	9 (1)	12 (9)	21 (13)	9 (2)	Compulsive Disorder
2 (2)	4 (5)	16 (7)	-	13 (5)	8 (2)	5 (3)	-	8 (2)	Panic disorder
118 (30)	102 (22)	152 (15)	157 (26)	112 (19)	124 (6)	123 (17)	118 (20)	123 (5)	**Any neurotic disorder**
8 (4)	-	4 (4)	11 (7)	6 (5)	4 (1)	2 (2)	11 (9)	4 (1)	**Functional psychoses**
61 (27)	82 (15)	67 (12)	113 (28)	96 (17)	72 (5)	87 (28)	99 (24)	75 (5)	**Alcohol dependence**
40 (21)	45 (16)	25 (8)	63 (23)	28 (11)	31 (3)	11 (5)	16 (6)	29 (3)	**Drug dependence**
									All adults
									Mixed anxiety and
61 (15)	73 (14)	92 (12)	95 (10)	66 (10)	77 (4)	73 (15)	70 (12)	77 (3)	depressive disorder
									Generalised
28 (6)	17 (6)	29 (7)	53 (8)	22 (6)	31 (2)	25 (7)	40 (6)	31 (2)	Anxiety Disorder
12 (8)	18 (5)	25 (5)	31 (7)	25 (6)	21 (2)	21 (5)	24 (8)	21 (1)	Depressive episode
20 (8)	5 (2)	9 (4)	11 (7)	12 (5)	11 (1)	10 (4)	10 (4)	11 (1)	All phobias
									Obsessive
6 (4)	7 (5)	11 (4)	21 (5)	7 (3)	11 (1)	13 (4)	26 (6)	12 (1)	Compulsive Disorder
5 (3)	5 (4)	13 (4)	2 (2)	16 (6)	9 (1)	10 (4)	-	8 (1)	Panic disorder
132 (27)	126 (14)	179 (16)	213 (26)	149 (17)	160 (5)	153 (17)	169 (18)	160 (5)	**Any neurotic disorder**
5 (2)	-	3 (2)	5 (3)	7 (4)	4 (1)	6 (4)	8 (3)	4 (1)	**Functional psychoses**
40 (13)	53 (11)	50 (9)	62 (16)	55 (13)	46 (3)	51 (13)	59 (7)	47 (3)	**Alcohol dependence**
27 (10)	28 (9)	22 (5)	34 (13)	23 (6)	23 (2)	14 (5)	19 (9)	22 (2)	**Drug dependence**

**Table 6.12 Prevalence of psychiatric disorders by locality and sex
(per thousand population)**

	Locality			All	
	Urban	Semi-rural	Rural		
	Rate per thousand in past week (SE)				
Women					
Mixed anxiety and depressive disorder	110 (6)	78 (8)	75 (15)	99 (5)	
Generalised Anxiety Disorder	38 (4)	29 (5)	19 (7)	34 (3)	
Depressive episode	29 (3)	16 (4)	15 (5)	25 (2)	
All phobias	16 (2)	12 (3)	9 (4)	14 (2)	
Obsessive-Compulsive Disorder	14 (2)	16 (4)	14 (4)	15 (2)	
Panic disorder	9 (2)	5 (2)	18 (7)	9 (1)	
Any neurotic disorder	216 (9)	156 (10)	150 (22)	195 (7)	
	Rate per thousand in past twelve months (SE)				
Functional psychoses	5 (1)	5 (2)	1 (1)	4 (1)	
Alcohol dependence	25 (3)	12 (3)	15 (6)	21 (2)	
Drug dependence	18 (3)	12 (4)	2 (1)	15 (2)	
	Rate per thousand in past week (SE)				
Men					
Mixed anxiety and depressive disorder	56 (5)	56 (8)	41 (10)	54 (4)	
Generalised Anxiety Disorder	31 (3)	23 (5)	21 (7)	28 (2)	
Depressive episode	19 (3)	18 (4)	6 (3)	17 (2)	
All phobias	9 (2)	3 (1)	3 (2)	7 (1)	
Obsessive-Compulsive Disorder	11 (2)	9 (3)	1 (1)	9 (2)	
Panic disorder	7 (2)	9 (4)	7 (4)	8 (2)	
Any neurotic disorder	133 (6)	117 (10)	78 (12)	123 (5)	
	Rate per thousand in past twelve months (SE)				
Functional psychoses	6 (1)	1 (1)	3 (4)	4 (1)	
Alcohol dependence	84 (6)	60 (7)	53 (15)	75 (5)	
Drug dependence	34 (4)	21 (6)	16 (6)	29 (3)	
	Rate per thousand in past week (SE)				
All adults					
Mixed anxiety and depressive disorder	83 (4)	67 (5)	57 (11)	77 (3)	
Generalised Anxiety Disorder	34 (2)	26 (3)	20 (5)	31 (2)	
Depressive episode	24 (2)	17 (3)	10 (3)	21 (1)	
All phobias	13 (2)	8 (2)	6 (3)	11 (1)	
Obsessive-Compulsive Disorder	13 (1)	12 (2)	7 (2)	12 (1)	
Panic disorder	8 (1)	7 (2)	12 (4)	8 (1)	
Any neurotic disorder	175 (6)	137 (7)	113 (15)	160 (5)	
	Rate per thousand in past twelve months (SE)				
Functional psychoses	5 (1)	3 (1)	2 (2)	4 (1)	
Alcohol dependence	54 (4)	36 (4)	34 (9)	47 (3)	
Drug dependence	26 (2)	16 (4)	9 (3)	22 (2)	

Table 6.13 Summary of significant odds ratios: psychiatric disorders

Asterisks represent increases or decreases (shaded cells) in odds.
For each variable the reference group is the first category listed.

	Neurotic disorders						Functional psychoses	Alcohol depen-dence	Drug dependence
	Depressive episode	Phobia	OCD	Panic disorder	GAD	Mixed anxiety/ depression			
Sex:									
Male									
Female					*	**		**	**
Age:									
16-24									
25-34			*		*			**	**
35-44					**			**	**
45-54					**			**	**
55-64			**		**	**		**	**
Ethnicity:									
White									
West Indian/African									
Asian or Oriental		*						**	
Other									
Qualifications:									
A level or higher									
GCSE/O level									
Other									
None	**						**		
Family unit type:									
Couple, no children									
Couple & child(ren)									
Lone parent & child(ren)	**					**		*	
One person only	**					**		**	**
Adult with parents									*
Adult with one parent								*	*
Employment status:									
Working full time									
Working part time		*					*		
Unemployed	**	**	**		**	**	*		**
Economically inactive	**	**	**		*		**		**
Accommodation:									
Detached									
Semi-detached									
Terraced								**	*
Flat or maisonette								**	**
Tenure:									
Owner occupier									
Renter				**	**	*	**		*
Locality:									
Semi-rural/rural									
Urban	*	*			*				

Significance *p<0.05
      **p<0.01

Table 6.14 Odds ratios of socio-demographic correlates of depressive episode

		Adjusted OR	(95% CI)
Age	16-24	1.00	....
	25-34	1.04	(0.65-1.67)
	35-44	1.22	(0.75-1.99)
	45-54	1.43	(0.88-2.34)
	55-64	0.63	(0.36-1.09)
Qualifications	A level or higher	1.00	....
	GCSE/O level	1.29	(0.87-1.90)
	Other	1.51	(0.94-2.41)
	None	1.67**	(1.15-2.42)
Family unit type	Couple, no children	1.00	....
	Couple & child(ren)	1.18	(0.76-1.81)
	Lone parent & child(ren)	2.60**	(1.60-4.26)
	One person only	2.32**	(1.53-3.50)
	Adult with parents	1.40	(0.67-2.96)
	Adult with one parent	1.46	(0.63-3.40)
Employment status	Working full time	1.00	....
	Working part time	1.50	(0.97-2.30)
	Unemployed	2.66**	(1.73-4.10)
	Economically inactive	2.87**	(2.03-4.11)
Locality	Semi-rural/rural	1.00	....
	Urban	1.38*	(1.01-1.88)

Significance: *   p<0.05
          ** p<0.01

Table 6.15 Odds ratios of socio-demographic correlates of phobia

		Adjusted OR	(95% CI)
Ethnicity	White	1.00	....
	West Indian or African	1.22*	(0.43-4.51)
	Asian or Oriental	2.34*	(1.07-5.12)
	Other	2.87	(0.88-9.26)
Employment status	Working full time	1.00	....
	Working part time	2.07*	(1.15-3.74)
	Unemployed	3.11**	(1.65-5.80)
	Economically inactive	3.28**	(2.05-5.26)
Locality	Semi-rural/rural	1.00	....
	Urban	1.66*	(1.04-2.67)

Significance: * p<0.05
          ** p<0.01

Table 6.16 Odds ratios of socio-demographic correlates of Obsessive-Compulsive Disorder

		Adjusted OR	(95% CI)
Age	**16-24**	1.00	....
	25-34	0.55*	(0.31-0.99)
	35-44	0.75	(0.42-1.35)
	45-54	0.60	(0.32-1.09)
	55-64	0.32**	(0.16-0.64)
Family unit type	**Couple, no children**	1.00	....
	Couple &child(ren)	0.62	(0.35-1.07)
	Lone parent & child(ren)	0.98	(0.41-1.63)
	One person only	1.38	(0.69-2.73)
	Adult with parents	0.38	(0.13-1.05)
	Adult with one parent	0.90	(0.14-1.00)
Employment status	**Working full time**	1.00	....
	Working part time	1.42	(0.82-2.46)
	Unemployed	2.11**	(1.20-3.74)
	Economically inactive	2.04**	(1.27-3.26)

Significance: * p<0.05
         ** p<0.01

Table 6.17 Odds ratios of socio-demographic correlates of Generalised Anxiety Disorder

		Adjusted OR	(95% CI)
Sex	**Male**	1.00	....
	Female	1.31*	(1.02-1.69)
Age	**16-24**	1.00	....
	25-34	1.92*	(1.15-3.19)
	35-44	2.67**	(1.60-4.44)
	45-54	3.47**	(2.10-5.81)
	55-64	3.20**	(1.92-5.31)
Employment status	**Working full time**	1.00	....
	Working part time	0.92	(0.64-1.34)
	Unemployed	2.19**	(1.53-3.10)
	Economically inactive	1.44*	(1.08-1.94)
Tenure	**Owner-occupier**	1.00	....
	Renter	1.42**	(1.12-1.80)
Locality	**Semi-rural/rural**	1.00	....
	Urban	1.30*	(1.01-1.67)

Significance: * p<0.05
         ** p<0.01

Table 6.18 Odds ratios of socio-demographic correlates of mixed anxiety and depressive disorder

		Adjusted OR	(95% CI)
Sex	Male	1.00	....
	Female	1.73**	(1.45-2.07)
Age	16-24	1.00	....
	25-34	1.03	(0.80-1.33)
	35-44	1.08	(0.82-1.43)
	45-54	0.92	(0.69-1.24)
	55-64	0.61**	(0.45-0.84)
Family unit type	Couple, no child(ren)	1.00	....
	Couple & child(ren)	1.09	(0.87-1.34)
	Lone parent & child(ren)	1.48**	(1.12-1.94)
	One person only	1.47**	(1.18-1.81)
	Adult with parents	0.63	(0.40-1.00)
	Adult with one parent	0.73	(0.42-1.26)
Employment status	Working full time	1.00	....
	Working part time	1.14	(0.92-1.41)
	Unemployed	1.73**	(1.34-2.24)
	Economically inactive	1.19	(0.97-1.49)
Accommodation	Detached	1.00	....
	Semi-detached	0.95	(0.75-1.20)
	Terraced	1.23	(0.98-1.56)
	Flat or maisonette	1.21	(0.92-1.59)
Tenure	Owner-occupier	1.00	....
	Renter	1.22*	(1.02-1.46)

Significance: * p<0.05
          ** p<0.01

Table 6.19 Odds ratios of socio-demographic correlates of panic disorder

		Adjusted OR	(95% CI)
Tenure	Owner-occupier	1.00	....
	Renter	2.46**	(1.60-3.79)

Significance: * p<0.05
          ** p<0.01

Table 6.20 Odds ratios of socio-demographic correlates of functional psychosis

		Adjusted OR	(95% CI)
Qualifications	A level or higher	1.00	....
	GCSE/O level	0.68	(0.34-1.34)
	Other	1.69	(0.29-1.67)
	None	1.27**	(0.13-0.59)
Employment status	Working full time	1.00	....
	Working part time	2.76*	(1.18-6.38)
	Unemployed	2.98*	(1.18-7.47)
	Economically inactive	3.46**	(1.66-7.20)
Tenure	Owner-occupier	1.00	....
	Renter	4.00**	(2.21-7.26)

Significance: * p<0.05
        ** p<0.01

Table 6.21 Odds ratios of socio-demographic correlates of alcohol dependence

		Adjusted OR	(95% CI)
Sex	Male	1.00	....
	Female	0.26**	(0.20-0.33)
Age	16-24	1.00	....
	25-34	0.63**	(0.48-0.82)
	35-44	0.39**	(0.28-0.55)
	45-54	0.27**	(0.18-0.39)
	55-64	0.09**	(0.05-0.16)
Ethnicity	White	1.00	....
	West Indian or African	0.67	(0.30-1.45)
	Asian or Oriental	0.13**	(0.03-0.52)
	Other	1.38	(0.60-3.14)
Family unit type	Couple, no children	1.00	....
	Couple & child(ren)	0.90	(0.64-1.25)
	Lone parent & child(ren)	1.74*	(1.08-2.77)
	One person only	2.08**	(1.52-2.84)
	Adult with parents	1.51	(0.98-2.32)
	Adult with one parent	1.79*	(1.09-2.92)
Accommodation	Detached	1.00	....
	Semi-detached	1.15	(0.79-1.67)
	Terraced	1.83**	(1.28-2.59)
	Flat or maisonette	2.15**	(1.49-3.13)

Significance: * p<0.05
        ** p<0.01

Table 6.22 Odds ratios of socio-demographic correlates of drug dependence

		Adjusted O.R.	(95% CI)
Sex	**Male**	1.00	....
	Female	0.64**	(0.46-0.89)
Age	**16-24**	1.00	....
	25-34	0.42**	(0.28-0.61)
	35-44	0.36**	(0.23-0.58)
	45-54	0.11**	(0.05-0.23)
	55-64	0.11**	(0.05-0.21)
Family unit type	**Couple, no children**	1.00	....
	Couple & child(ren)	1.04	(0.55-1.99)
	Lone parent& child(ren)	1.42	(0.69-2.93)
	One person only	2.95**	(1.67-5.20)
	Adult with parents	2.38*	(0.20-4.74)
	Adult with one parent	2.43*	(1.13-5.23)
Employment status	**Working full time**	1.00	....
	Working part time	1.69	(0.99-2.86)
	Unemployed	3.80**	(2.55-5.60)
	Economically inactive	2.34**	(1.55-3.67)
Accommodation	**Detached**	1.00	
	Semi-detached	1.38	(0.72-2.63)
	Terraced	2.09*	(1.12-3.92)
	Flat or maisonette	2.50**	(0.29-4.89)
Tenure	**Owner-occupier**	1.00	
	Renter	1.57*	(1.10-2.23)

Significance: *   p<0.05
               ** p<0.01

Table 6.23 Odds ratios for the co-occurence of disorders derived from the revised Clinical Interview Schedule (CIS - R)

Diagnosis 1	Diagnosis 2	Odds ratio*	(95% CI)
Depresive episode	Obsessive Compulsive Disorder	26.79	(18.25-39.26)
Phobia	Obsessive Compulsive Disorder	23.94	(15.85-36.09)
Depresive episode	Generalised Anxiety Disorder	14.76	(10.89-19.99)
Generalised Anxiety Disorder	Obsessive Compulsive Disorder	15.90	(11.20-22.54)
Depressive episode	Phobia	17.15	(11.63-25.23)

* These represent the odds of diagnosis 2, given diagnosis 1.

Appendix A Sampling, non-response and weighting

A.1 Sampling of individuals within households

One adult aged 16 to 64 years was interviewed in each household. This was done in preference to interviewing all eligible adults because:

(a) it helped interviewers to conduct the interview in privacy and thereby obtain more reliable information;

(b) individuals within households will tend to be similar to each other and where households differ markedly from one another, the resultant clustering can lead to a substantial increase in standard errors around survey estimates. By selecting only one person in each household, this clustering effect was overcome;

(c) it reduced the interviewing burden placed on the household.

Selection procedure

In households where there was more than one person aged 16 to 64, one had to be selected at random for interview, ensuring that all household members who were eligible for the survey had the same chance of being selected.

The selection procedure carried out at the household was as follows:

(i)   The interviewers listed all household members and their ages. They sorted the household members who were aged 16 to 64 and hence were eligible for the survey into descending order of age. Each eligible person was assigned a person number.

(ii) The person to be interviewed was then defined by reference to a selection table which was printed on a set of reference cards.

(iii) The cards indicate which one of the eligible people should be selected for a given address depending on the number of eligible people in the household.

The selection table was based on those designed by

Kish, which gave a close approximation to the proper fractional representation of each eligible adult in the household for up to six adults[1]. For this survey, selection tables for up to 8 eligible adults were used and a different set of possible selections were shown for each of the 90 addresses in each postal sector.

In theory this meant that in households with 9 or more eligible people some people would not get a chance of selection. In practice no households as large as these were found on this survey.

Often the person who had been selected for interview was not the person who was giving the household details, and so interviewers made arrangements to interview the selected person.

References

1. Kish L. *Survey Sampling*. J Wiley & Sons Ltd London 1965.

A.2 Characteristics of non - respondents

Normally there is very little information about people who do not respond to surveys – the fact they do not respond means it is difficult to find out anything about them. Where households could not be contacted or refused to take part, interviewers were instructed to find out about the members of the household and note their age and sex. This sometimes involved asking neighbours for estimates where there was complete non-response from a household.

In households which had agreed to take part but where the person who was selected at random for the survey did not respond, either because they refused or because they could not be contacted, interviewers were usually able to collect this information from other members of the household.

Knowing the age and sex of people in responding and non-responding households, we can examine the characteristics of non responders to see whether they are significantly different to responders and whether their omission substantially changed the composition of the sample.

What such analysis can not do is estimate any non-response bias associated with psychiatric morbidity itself. Interviewers therefore also recorded the reasons which people gave for refusing to take part.

Two per cent of eligible households refused direct to OPCS headquarters to take part in the survey. Wherever possible, information about the household and the reasons for the refusal were also obtained.

Non-response and household size

There was an association between the size of the household and its likelihood of co-operating. Household size was defined as the number of people aged 16 to 64 in the household who were thereby eligible for the survey. Household size was not known for 12 % of households. Households with just one adult aged 16 to 64 were more likely to be non-responding than co-operating households. Differential non-response according to household size was one of the factors which was taken into account when weighting the survey data and is described in more detail in section A.3.

Non-response and age and sex of household members

One might expect that certain types of people as described by their sex and age-group were more likely to have been missed out of this survey because of non-response. Table A2.1 shows the ages of the household members for men and women by whether they were in co-operating or non-responding households, for members of households where the age and sex was known.

For men, there was very little difference in the proportions in the various five-year age bands between the co-operating households and the non-responding ones, although it appears that men aged 40 to 44 were over-represented in non-responding households, but men aged 45 to 49 were proportionally more likely to be in co-operating households than non-responding ones.

There were proportionally fewer women aged 16 to 19 in non-responding households compared with co-operating ones, but proportionally more women aged 50 to 54 in non-responding households. The final database also showed age-sex differences from the population, and weighting was carried out which

Table A2.1 Age of household members by response to survey and sex

Members of households where age and sex was known

Age	Response		All
	Co-operating	Non-responding	
	%	%	%
Women			
16-19	8	5	8
20-24	11	9	10
25-29	12	12	12
30-34	12	13	12
35-39	11	12	11
40-44	10	10	10
45-49	11	10	11
50-54	9	12	9
55-59	8	8	8
60-64	8	10	8
Base	*11268*	*1549*	*12817*
Men			
16-19	8	7	8
20-24	10	10	10
25-29	12	11	12
30-34	12	12	12
35-39	11	10	11
40-44	10	13	11
45-49	12	9	11
50-54	9	10	9
55-59	8	9	8
60-64	8	8	8
Base	*10950*	*1548*	*12498*

compensated for these differences. This is described in section A.3 below.

Reasons for refusing to co-operate

There is evidence that people who refuse to take part in surveys about mental health are more likely to have a mental health problem than those who co-operate. Goldberg (1988) states:

> "There is evidence to suggest that physically ill people may be more likely to respond....while the converse may be true for people with psychiatric disorders" (p62)

Table A2.2 shows that the most frequently given reasons for refusals were that households or selected informants could not be bothered, were too busy, did not believe in surveys or having their privacy disturbed. Only one in nine of the households or selected informants refused because of 'personal problems'.

Table A2.2 Reasons for refusals *

	%
Could not be bothered	36
Genuinely too busy	27
Did not believe in surveys	25
Invasion of privacy	22
Personal problems	11
Disliked survey matter	9
Anti-government	9
Worried about confidentiality	5
Too sick	4
Base	*1641*

* Percentages add to more than 100% because some
informants gave more than one reason.

A.3 Weighting for non-response and household size

Weighting occurred in three steps. First, weights
were applied to allow for non-response (refusals and
non-contacts) associated with household size.
Second, sample weights were applied to take account
of the different probabilities of selecting informants
in different sized households. Third, all respondents
were weighted up to represent the age-sex structure
of the total national population living in private
households.

*(i) Weighting to correct for different response rates
in different sizes of household*

Information on the number of people in the household and their age and sex was collected by OPCS
interviewers from households who were eligible for
inclusion in the survey but which refused or did not
respond. Thus, the household composition of non-
responding households was known for all sampled
eligible addresses and could be used in weighting. As
indicated in section A2 the household size (based on
number of individuals aged 16 to 64) of 1487 cases
was unknown. The household size of these cases was
determined by examining the interviewer's record of
the calls they made and their outcome. This indicated
that the majority of such cases were in household
size 2.

The association between household size and response
is shown in Table A3.1. Non-response is shown
separately for refusals and non-contacts at the
sampling stage.

Household size categories 4 to 7 were subsequently
collapsed into one category to give four household
size categories from which to calculate the weights.

Table A3.1 Association between response and household size

House-hold size	Response			
	Refusal	Non contact	Inter-view	Row total
1	535	204	2708	3447
2	907	687	5599	7093
3	138	60	1273	1471
4	56	27	528	611
5	5	2	87	94
6	0	1	10	11
7	0	0	3	3
Total	1641	981	10108	12730

(Loglinear modelling of the effect of household size
on non-response had indicated that there was no
improvement gained by calculating seven as
opposed to four separate final weights for non-
response.)

Non-response therefore varied with household size
when household size ranged from 1 to 4. Weights
were derived for each category of household size
using the formula 1.

$$weight = \frac{r}{r_c} \qquad \text{Formula 1}$$

where r =overall response rate
and r_c = response rate for a category of household
size.

r (overall response rate) works out at 0.79. The
household weights, r_{c1-4}, are shown in Table A3.2.

Table A3.2 Household weights for each household size

Household size	r_c		Household - weight (Weight 1)	
1	2708/3447	0.79/0.79	= 1.00	
2	5599/7093	0.79/0.78	= 1.01	
3	1273/1471	0.79/0.87	= 0.9	
4+	628/719	0.79/0.87	= 0.91	

Sample weights were next calculated to weight for
the different probabilities of selecting an informant
in different sized households (Table A3.3).

The sample data were then weighted by the
resulting non-response weight before calculating its
age-sex distribution.

Table A3.3 Non-response weights for each household size

Household size	Weight 1	Sample (weight 2)	Non-response (weight 3= 1* weight 2)
1	1.00	1	1.00
2	1.01	2	2.02
3	0.91	3	2.73
4+	0.91	4	3.64

(ii) Calculating weights to correct for non-response bias associated with age and sex

The next step in the weighting process involved calculating weights to correct for non-response bias associated with age and sex. First, the age-sex distribution of the sample (weighted as described above) was calculated, with age grouped into five-year bands. This was then compared with the age-sex distribution of the population (excluding individuals in institutions), from population projections from the 1981 Census to produce the age-sex weights shown in Table A3.4.

The final weight applied to the sample is the product of three sets of weights:

1. The household size weight. This corresponds to Weight 1 in Table A3.3, with a range of weights covering the full range of household sizes from 1 to 7 (Table A3.5).

2. The sample weights. These are as shown in Table A3.3, ranging from 1 to 7 to cover the full range of household sizes.

3. The age-sex weights (Table A3.4).

For example, applying the product of the three weights would give a weight for a female aged 16-19 in household size 1 of 1.16 (i.e., 1.00*1.00*1.16).

After the weights were applied the weighted sample size differed from the actual (pre-weighting) sample size. A final weighting factor (Formula 2) was therefore applied to correct the change in the base. This returned the weighted sample size to its original size.

$$\frac{\text{Unweighted sample size}}{\text{weighted sample size}} \quad \text{Formula 2}$$

Table A3.4 Age-sex weights

	Population proportion	Sample proportion	Age-sex weight
Men			
16-19	3.8	3.4	1.12
20-24	5.9	5.0	1.18
25-29	6.6	5.6	1.18
30-34	6.0	6.0	1.00
35-39	5.3	5.3	1.00
40-44	5.3	4.9	1.08
45-49	5.2	5.2	1.00
50-54	4.2	4.4	0.96
55-59	4.0	4.3	0.93
60-64	3.8	4.0	0.95
Women			
16-19	3.7	3.2	1.16
20-24	5.7	5.0	1.14
25-29	6.4	6.4	1.00
30-34	5.9	6.1	0.97
35-39	5.3	5.8	0.91
40-44	5.4	5.8	0.93
45-49	5.2	6.3	0.83
50-54	4.2	4.8	0.88
55-59	4.0	4.0	1.00
60-64	4.0	4.5	0.89

Population proportions were obtained from the OPCS Population Estimates Unit and Population Statistics Branch, General Register Office for Scotland.

Table A3.5 Household size weights for household sizes 1 to 7

Household size	Household size weight
1	1.00
2	1.01
3	0.91
4	0.92
5	0.85
6	0.87
7	0.79

References

1. Goldberg, D., and Williams, P., (1988). *A Users Guide to the General Health Questionnaire*, NFER-NELSON.

Appendix B Psychiatric measurement

B.1 Calculation of CIS-R symptom scores

Fatigue

Scores relate to fatigue or feeling tired or lacking in energy in the past week.
Score one for each of:
- Symptom present on four days or more
- Symptom present for more than three hours in total on any day
- Subject had to push him/herself to get things done on at least one occasion
- Symptom present when subject doing things he/she enjoys or used to enjoy at least once

Sleep problems

Scores relate to problems with getting to sleep, or otherwise, with sleeping more than is usual for the subject in the past week.
Score one for each of:
- Had problems with sleep for four nights or more
- Spent at least ¼ hours trying to get to sleep on the night with least sleep
- Spent at least 1 hour trying to get to sleep on the night with least sleep
- Spent three hours or more trying to get to sleep on four nights or more
- Slept for at least ¼ hours longer than usual for subject on any night
- Slept for at least 1 hour longer than usual for subject on any night
- Slept for more than three hours longer than usual for subject on four nights or more

Irritability

Scores relate to feelings of irritability, being short-tempered or angry in the past week.
Score one for each of:
- Symptom present for four days or more
- Symptom present for more than one hour on any day
- Wanted to shout at someone (even if subject had not actually shouted)
- Had arguments, rows or quarrels or lost temper with someone and felt it was unjustified on at least one occasion

Worry

Scores relate to subject's experience of worry in the past week, other than worry about physical Health.
Score one for each of:
- Symptom present on four or more days

- Has been worrying too much in view of circumstances
- Symptom has been very unpleasant
- Symptom lasted over three hours in total on any day

Depression

Applies to subjects who felt sad, miserable or depressed or unable to enjoy or take an interest in things as much as usual, in the past week. Scores relate to the subject's experience in the past week.
Score one for each of:
- Unable to enjoy or take an interest in things as much as usual
- Symptom present on four days or more
- Symptom lasted for more than three hours in total on any day
- When sad, miserable or depressed subject did not become happier when something nice happened, or when in company

Depressive ideas

Applies to subjects who had a score of 1 for depression. Scores relate to experience in the past week.
Score one for each of:
- Felt guilty or blamed him/herself at least once when things went wrong when it had not been his/her fault
- Felt not as good as other people
- Felt hopeless
- Felt that life isn't worth living
- Thought of killing him/herself

Anxiety

Scores relate to feeling generally anxious, nervous or tense in the past week. These feelings were not the result of a phobia.
Score one for each of:
- Symptom present on four or more days
- Symptom had been very unpleasant
- When anxious, nervous or tense, had one or more of following symptoms:
    heart racing or pounding
    hands sweating or shaking
    feeling dizzy
    difficulty getting breath
    butterflies in stomach
    dry mouth
    nausea or feeling as though he/she wanted to vomit
- Symptom present for more than three hours in total on any one day

Obsessions

Scores relate to the subject's experience of having repetitive unpleasant thoughts or ideas in the past week.

Score one for each of:

- Symptom present on four or more days
- Tried to stop thinking any of these thoughts
- Became upset or annoyed when had these thoughts
- Longest episode of the symptom was $\frac{1}{4}$ hour or longer

Concentration and forgetfulness

Scores relate to the subject's experience of concentration problems and forgetfulness in the past week.

Score one for each of:

- Symptoms present for four days or more
- Could not always concentrate on a TV programme, read a newspaper article or talk to someone without mind wandering
- Problems with concentration stopped subject from getting on with things he/she used to do or would have liked to do
- Forgot something important

Somatic symptoms

Scores relate to the subject's experience in the past week of any ache, pain or discomfort which was brought on or made worse by feeling low, anxious or stressed.

Score one for each of:

- Symptom present for four days or more
- Symptom lasted more than three hours on any day
- Symptom had been very unpleasant
- Symptom bothered subject when doing something interesting

Compulsions

Scores relate to the subject's experience of doing things over again when subject had already done them in the past week.

Score one for each of:

- Symptom present on four days or more
- Subject tried to stop repeating behaviour
- Symptom made subject upset or annoyed with him/herself
- Repeated behaviour three or more times when it had already been done

Phobias

Scores relate to subject's experience of phobias or avoidance in the past week

Score one for each of:

- Felt nervous/anxious about a situation or thing four or more times

- On occasions when felt anxious, nervous or tense, had one or more of following symptoms:
    heart racing or pounding
    hands sweating or shaking
    feeling dizzy
    difficulty getting breath
    butterflies in stomach
    dry mouth
    nausea or feeling as though he/she wanted to vomit
- Avoided situation or thing at least once because it would have made subject anxious, nervous or tense
- Avoided situation or thing four times or more because it would have made subject anxious, nervous or tense

Worry about physical health

Scores relate to experience of the symptom in the past week.

Score one for each of:

- Symptom present on four days or more
- Subject felt he/she had been worrying too much in view of actual health
- Symptom had been very unpleasant
- Subject could not be distracted by doing something else

Panic

Applies to subjects who felt anxious, nervous or tense in the past week and the scores relate to the resultant feelings of panic, or of collapsing and losing control in the past week.

Score one for each of:

- Symptom experienced once
- Symptom experienced more than once
- Symptom had been very unpleasant or unbearable
- An episode lasted longer than 10 minutes

B.2 Algorithms to produce ICD-10 psychiatric disorders

The mental disorders reported in Chapter 6 were produced from the CIS-R schedule which is described in Chapter 2 and reproduced in Appendix C. The production of the six categories of disorder shown in these tables occurred in 3 stages: first, the informants' responses to the CIS-R were used to produce specific ICD-10 diagnoses of neurosis. This was done by applying the algorithms described below. Second, these specific neurotic disorders plus psychosis were arranged hierarchically and the 'highest' disorder assumed precedence. The actual precedence rules are described below. Finally, the range of ICD-10 diagnoses were grouped together to produce categories used in the calculation of prevalence.

It should be noted that as a result of the hierarchical coding described above, the diagnoses of the six neurotic disorders and the category of functional psychosis are exclusive: an individual included in the prevalence rates for one neurotic or psychotic disorder is not included in calculation of the rate for any other neurotic or psychotic disorder. This does not apply to the diagnoses of alcohol and drug dependence.

Algorithms for production of ICD-10 diagnoses of neurosis from the CIS-R ('scores' refer to CIS-R scores)

F32.00 Mild depressive episode without somatic symptoms

1. Symptom duration ≥ 2 weeks

2. *Two or more from:*
   - depressed mood
   - loss of interest
   - fatigue

3. *Two or three from:*
   - reduced concentration
   - reduced self-esteem
   - ideas of guilt
   - pessimism about future
   - suicidal ideas or acts
   - disturbed sleep
   - diminished appetite

4. Social impairment

5. *Fewer than four from:*
   - lack of normal pleasure /interest
   - loss of normal emotional reactivity
   - a.m. waking ≥ 2 hours early
   - loss of libido
   - diurnal variation in mood
   - diminished appetite
   - loss of ≥ 5% body weight
   - psychomotor agitation
   - psychomotor retardation

F32.01 Mild depressive episode with somatic symptoms

1. Symptom duration ≥ 2 weeks

2. *Two or more from:*
   - depressed mood
   - loss of interest
   - fatigue

3. *Two or three from:*
   - reduced concentration
   - reduced self-esteem
   - ideas of guilt
   - pessimism about future
   - suicidal ideas or acts
   - disturbed sleep
   - diminished appetite

4. Social impairment

5. *Four or more from:*
   - lack of normal pleasure /interest
   - loss of normal emotional reactivity
   - a.m. waking ≥ 2 hours early
   - loss of libido
   - diurnal variation in mood
   - diminished appetite
   - loss of 5% body weight
   - psychomotor agitation
   - psychomotor retardation

F32.10 Moderate depressive episode without somatic symptoms

1. Symptom duration ≥2 weeks

2. *Two or more* from:
   - depressed mood
   - loss of interest
   - fatigue

3. *Four or more* from:
   - reduced concentration
   - reduced self-esteem
   - ideas of guilt
   - pessimism about future
   - suicidal ideas or acts
   - disturbed sleep
   - diminished appetite

4. Social impairment

5. *Fewer than four* from:
   - lack of normal pleasure/interest
   - loss of normal emotional reactivity
   - a.m. waking ≥ 2 hours early
   - loss of libido
   - diurnal variation in mood
   - diminished appetite
   - loss of ≥ 5% body weight
   - psychomotor agitation
   - psychomotor retardation

F32.11 Moderate depressive episode with somatic symptoms

1. Symptom duration ≥2 weeks

2. *Two or more* from:
   - depressed mood
   - loss of interest
   - fatigue

3. *Four or more* from:
   - reduced concentration
   - reduced self-esteem
   - ideas of guilt
   - pessimism about future
   - suicidal ideas or acts
   - disturbed sleep
   - diminished appetite

4. Social impairment

5. *Four or more* from:
   - lack of normal pleasure /interest
   - loss of normal emotional reactivity
   - a.m. waking ≥2 hours early
   - loss of libido
   - diurnal variation in mood
   - diminished appetite
   - loss of ≥ 5% body weight
   - psychomotor agitation
   - psychomotor retardation

F32.2 Severe depressive episode

1. *All three* from:
   - depressed mood
   - loss of interest
   - fatigue

2. *Four or more* from:
   - reduced concentration
   - reduced self-esteem
   - ideas of guilt
   - pessimism about future
   - suicidal ideas or acts
   - disturbed sleep
   - diminished appetite

3. Social impairment

4. *Four or more* from:
   - lack of normal pleasure /interest
   - loss of normal emotional reactivity
   - a.m. waking ≥ 2 hours early
   - loss of libido
   - diurnal variation in mood
   - diminished appetite

   - loss of ≥ 5% body weight
   - psychomotor agitation
   - psychomotor retardation

F40.00 Agoraphobia without panic disorder
1. Fear of open spaces and related aspects: crowds, distance from home, travelling alone
2. Social impairment
3. Avoidant behaviour must be prominent feature
4. Overall phobia score ≥ 2
5. No panic attacks

F40.01 Agoraphobia with panic disorder
1. Fear of open spaces and related aspects: crowds, distance from home, travelling alone
2. Social impairment
3. Avoidant behaviour must be prominent feature
4. Overall phobia score ≥ 2
5. Panic disorder (overall panic score ≥ 2)

F40.1 Social phobias
1. Fear of scrutiny by other people: eating or speaking in public etc.
2. Social impairment
3. Avoidant behaviour must be prominent feature
4. Overall phobia score ≥ 2

F40.2 Specific (isolated) phobias
1. Fear of specific situations or things, e.g. animals, insects, heights, blood, flying, etc.
2. Social impairment
3. Avoidant behaviour must be prominent feature
4. Overall phobia score ≥ 2

F41.0 Panic disorder
1. Criteria for phobic disorders not met
2. Recent panic attacks
3. Anxiety-free between attacks
4. Overall panic score ≥ 2

F41.1 Generalised Anxiety Disorder
1. Duration ≥ 6 months
2. Free-floating anxiety
3. Autonomic overactivity
4. Overall anxiety score ≥ 2

F41.2 Mixed anxiety and depressive disorder
1. (Sum of scores for each CIS-R section) ≥ 12
2. Criteria for other categories not met

F42 Obsessive-Compulsive Disorder
1. Duration ≥ 2 weeks
2. At least one act/thought resisted
3. Social impairment
4. Overall scores:
   obsession score=4, or
   compulsion score=4, or
   obsession+compulsion scores ≥6

Hierarchical organisation of psychiatric disorders

The following rules (see table below) were used to allocate individuals who received more than one diagnosis of neurosis to the appropriate category.

Grouping neurotic and psychotic disorders into broad categories

The final step was to group some of the diagnoses into broad diagnostic categories prior to analysis.

Depressive episode

F32.00 and F32.01 were grouped to produce mild depressive episode (i.e. with or without somatic symptoms). F32.10 and F32.11 were similarly grouped to produce moderate depressive episode. Mild depressive episode, moderate depressive episode and Severe depressive episode (F32.2) were then combined to produce the final category of depressive episode.

Phobias

The ICD-10 phobic diagnoses F40.00, F40.01, F40.1 and F40.2, were combined into one category of phobia.

This produced six categories of neurosis for analysis:

> Mixed anxiety and depressive disorder
> Generalised Anxiety Disorder
> Depressive episode
> All phobias
> Obsessive Compulsive Disorder
> Panic disorder

B.3 Psychosis

The category of functional psychosis shown in Tables 6.1 to 6.12 actually subsumes five sub-categories of psychosis: four categories (schizophrenia, manic episode, bipolar affective disorder and other functional psychosis) were derived from the SCAN interview by clinicians. The fifth category constitutes diagnoses of psychosis made on the basis of data collected by OPCS interviewers, as described in Chapter 6.

B.4 Assessing alcohol and drug dependence

Questions relating to alcohol and drug dependence were included in a self-completion questionnaire (Appendix C) which were asked of all informants, i.e. irrespective of whether they were reported as having a mental health problem on the assessment schedules.

Alcohol dependence

The twelve questions on alcohol dependence were taken from the National Alcohol Survey carried out in the USA in 1984[1]. An anglicised version was created to measure the three components of dependence: loss of control, symptomatic behaviour and binge drinking.

Disorder 1	Disorder 2	Priority
Depressive episode (any severity)	Phobia	Depressive episode (any severity)
Depressive episode (mild)	OCD	OCD
Depressive episode (moderate)	OCD	Depressive episode (moderate)
Depressive episode (severe)	OCD	Depressive episode (severe)
Depressive episode (mild)	Panic disorder	Panic disorder
Depressive episode (moderate)	Panic disorder	Depressive episode (moderate)
Depressive episode (any severity)	GAD	Depressive episode (any severity)
Phobia (any)	OCD	OCD
Agoraphobia	GAD	Agoraphobia
Social phobia	GAD	Social phobia
Specific phobia	GAD	GAD
Panic disorder	OCD	Panic disorder
OCD	GAD	OCD
Panic disorder	GAD	Panic disorder

GAD = Generalised Anxiety Disorder OCD = Obsessive–Compulsive Disorder

Loss of control

Score one for positive response to each of:

1. Once I started drinking it was difficult for me to stop before I became completely drunk

2. I sometimes kept on drinking after I had promised myself not to.

3. I deliberately tried to cut down or stop drinking, but I was unable to do so.

4. Sometimes I have needed a drink so badly that I could not think of anything else.

Symptomatic behaviour

Score one for positive response to each of:

1. I have skipped a number of regular meals while drinking.

2. I have often had an alcoholic drink the first thing when I got up in the morning.

3. I have had a strong drink in the morning to get over the previous night's drinking.

4. I have woken up the next day not being able to remember some of the things I had done while drinking.

5. My hand shook a lot in the morning after drinking.

6. I need more alcohol than I used to get the same effect as before.

7. Sometimes I have woken up during the night or early morning sweating all over because of drinking.

Binge drinking

Score one for:

1. I have stayed drunk for several days at a time.

Although Room[1] originally had 13 items the same method of classifying severity of dependence was chosen:

0 items affirmed = no problem
1-2 items affirmed= minimal problem
3 or more items affirmed = at least a moderate problem
4 or more items affirmed = problem at a high level

For the tables in this report alcohol dependence refers to anyone with at least a moderate problem, that is, with a score of 3 or more.

Drug dependence

Questions on drug use and dependence were taken from the ECA[2] study. In the current study informants were shown a list of ten types of drug (with examples of their most common names) and had to answer questions by referring to this list (Appendix C). Five questions focused on drug dependence.

1. Have you ever used any one of these drugs every day for two weeks or more in the past twelve months?

2. In the past twelve months have you used any one of these drugs to the extent that you felt like you needed it or were dependent on it?

3. In the past twelve months, have you tried to cut down on any drugs but found you could not do it?

4. In the past twelve months did you find that you needed larger amounts of these drugs to get an effect, or that you could no longer get high on the amount you used to use?

5. In the past twelve months have you had withdrawal symptoms such as feeling sick because you stopped or cut down on any of these drugs?

A positive response to any of the above five questions was regarded as having at least some level of drug dependence and this measure (along with alcohol dependence) is included in the bottom half of the tables in Chapter 6.

References

1. Clark, W.B. and Hilton, M.E. (eds) (1991). *Alcohol in America: drinking practices and problems.* State University of New York Press, Albany.

2. Robins, L.N. and Regier, D.A. (1991). *Psychiatric disorders in America: the Epidemiological Catchment Area Study.* The Free Press (Macmillan Inc.), New York.

Appendix C The survey documents

N1361   Sift Schedule   **A**

IN CONFIDENCE

Stick serial number label

H'hld [ ]

Date of Interview [ ][ ] [ ][ ] **9** **3**

Interviewer's Name _____

Auth no. [ ][ ][ ]

1. Interviewer: code at start of interview

Record from observation

Urban	1	
Semi-rural	2	→ **Go to question 2, page 2**
Rural	3	

Interviewer: code at end of interview

Eligible for long interview (Subject interview)

Code all that apply:

Coded 1 at 11(b), page 6	01
Coded 1 at 13(b), page 7	02
Coded 1 at 14(b), page 7	03
Coded 1 at 17(b), page 8	04
Screened positive (coded 1) at P6, page 45	05
Has a score of 12 or more on check card	06

→ **Go to Schedule B (Yellow)**

Eligible for long interview (Proxy interview)

Code all that apply:

Coded 1 or 2 at Q2(b), page 46	07
Coded 1 at Q4(b), page 47	08
Coded 1 at Q5(b), page 47	09
Coded 1 or 2 at Q8(b), page 48	10

→ **Go to Schedule B (Yellow)**

Others - eligible for short interview

Subject interview	11
Proxy interview	12

→ **Go to Schedule C (Green)**

2 Details of all household members

Person no. Ring	Relationship to selected informant	Sex M F	Age now	Marital Status M C S W D Sep	Family unit	(a) Racial or ethnic group
(01)	Selected informant	OFF USE 00 — 1 2		1 2 3 4 5 6	(1)	
02		1 2		1 2 3 4 5 6		
03		1 2		1 2 3 4 5 6		
04		1 2		1 2 3 4 5 6		
05		1 2		1 2 3 4 5 6		
06		1 2		1 2 3 4 5 6		
07		1 2		1 2 3 4 5 6		
08		1 2		1 2 3 4 5 6		
09		1 2		1 2 3 4 5 6		
10		1 2		1 2 3 4 5 6		

(a) Ask or record

To which of the groups listed on this card do you consider you/(PERSON) belong(s)?
Record answer in column (a) of household box.

[Show card 1]

White	1
Black - Caribbean	2
Black - African	3
Black - Other	4
Indian	5
Pakistani	6
Bangladeshi	7
Chinese	8
None of these	9

Household check :

Code from household box

Interviewer code: number of children (aged under 16) →

Interviewer code: number of adults aged 16 to 64 →

Interviewer code: number of adults aged 65 or more →

Type of accommodation and tenure

4 Interviewer code

Type of accommodation occupied by this household:

Code from observation, if in doubt ask informant

Whole house, bungalow, detached	1
Whole house, bungalow, semi-detached	2
Whole house, bungalow, terraced/end of terrace	3
Purpose built flat/maisonette in block	4
Converted flat or maisonette in house	5
Room in house or block/bedsit	6
Other	7

5 Does your household own or rent this house/flat/room?

Owns	1 → (a)
Rents	2 → (b)
Rent free	3

(a) Is this house/flat:

Running prompt

Owned outright	1
or is it being bought with a mortgage or loan?	2 → 6

(b) Who is it rented from?
(Who is it provided by?)

Organisations:

Local authority/New Town	1
Housing association/co-operative or charitable trust	2
Property company	3
Employer	4
Other organisation	5

Individuals:

Relative or friend	6
Employer	7
Other individual	8

6 Ask or record

How many bedrooms does your household have, including bedsitting rooms and spare bedrooms?

Exclude bedrooms converted to other uses

1 - 8 Enter No	
9 or more	9

7   Does your household have a telephone in your (part of the) accommodation?

Shared telephones located in public hallways to be included only if this household is responsible for paying account.

Yes 1
No 2

8   Is there a car or van normally available for use by you (or any members of your household)?

INCLUDE: Any provided by employers if normally available for private use by informant or members of the household.

Yes .... 1 → (a)
No .... 2 → 9

(a) Is there one or more than one?

Prompt as necessary

1 1
2 2
3 or more 3

9   Interviewer check:

Interview to continue with subject ...... 1 → 10
Interview to continue with proxy .... 2 → Section Q, page 46

General health

10   How is your health in general? Would you say it was. . .

Running prompt

very good 1
good 2
fair 3
bad 4
or very bad? 5

11   Do you have any long-standing illness, disability or infirmity? By long-standing I mean anything that has troubled you over a period of time or that is likely to affect you over a period of time?

Yes .... 1 → (a)
No .... 2 → 12

(a) What is the matter with you?

Try and obtain a medical diagnosis or establish main symptoms

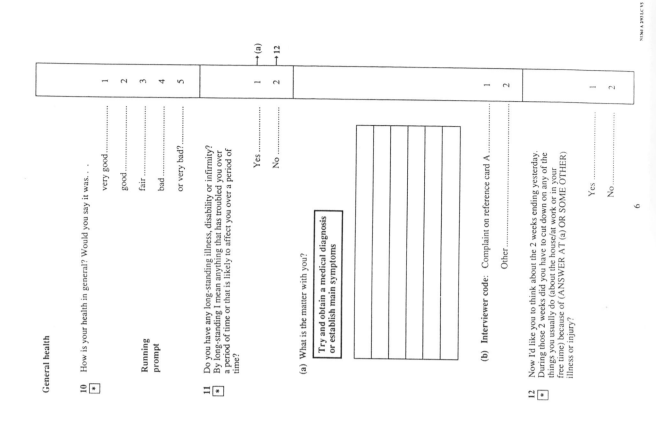

(b) Interviewer code: Complaint on reference card A 1
Other 2

12   Now I'd like you to think about the 2 weeks ending yesterday. During those 2 weeks did you have to cut down on any of the things you usually do (about the house/at work or in your free time) because of (ANSWER AT (a) OR SOME OTHER) illness or injury?

Yes 1
No 2

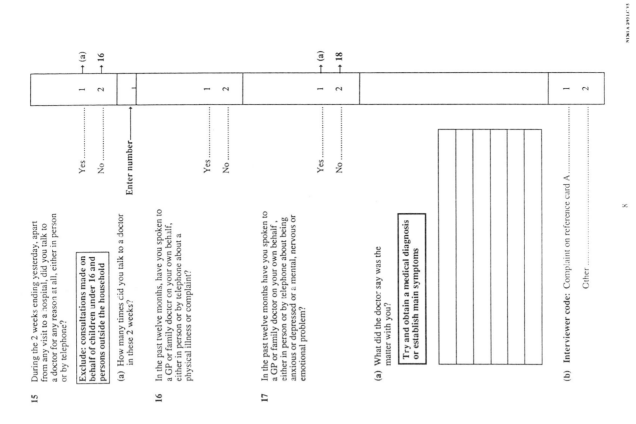

15 During the 2 weeks ending yesterday, apart from any visit to a hospital, did you talk to a doctor for any reason at all, either in person or by telephone?

Yes .... 1 → (a)
No .... 2 → 16

Exclude: consultations made on behalf of children under 16 and persons outside the household

(a) How many times did you talk to a doctor in these 2 weeks?

Enter number

16 In the past twelve months, have you spoken to a GP or family doctor on your own behalf, either in person or by telephone about a physical illness or complaint?

Yes 1
No 2

17 In the past twelve months have you spoken to a GP or family doctor on your own behalf, either in person or by telephone about being anxious or depressed or a mental, nervous or emotional problem?

Yes .... 1 → (a)
No .... 2 → 18

(a) What did the doctor say was the matter with you?

Try and obtain a medical diagnosis or establish main symptoms

(b) Interviewer code: Complaint on reference card A 1

Other 2

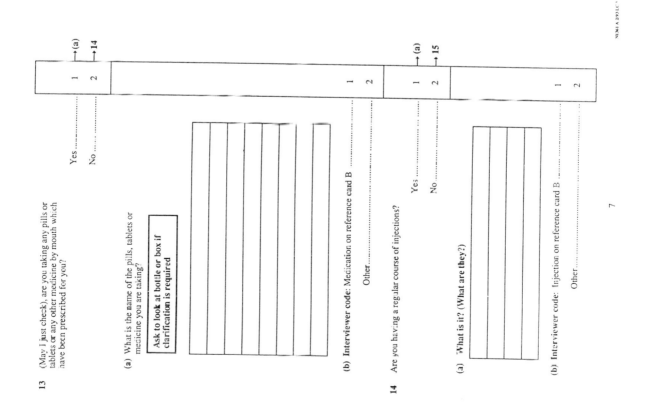

13 (May I just check), are you taking any pills or tablets or any other medicine by mouth which have been prescribed for you?

Yes .... 1 → (a)
No .... 2 → 14

(a) What is the name of the pills, tablets or medicine you are taking?

Ask to look at bottle or box if clarification is required

(b) Interviewer code: Medication on reference card B 1

Other 2

14 Are you having a regular course of injections?

Yes .... 1 → (a)
No .... 2 → 15

(a) What is it? (What are they?)

(b) Interviewer code: Injection on reference card B 1

Other 2

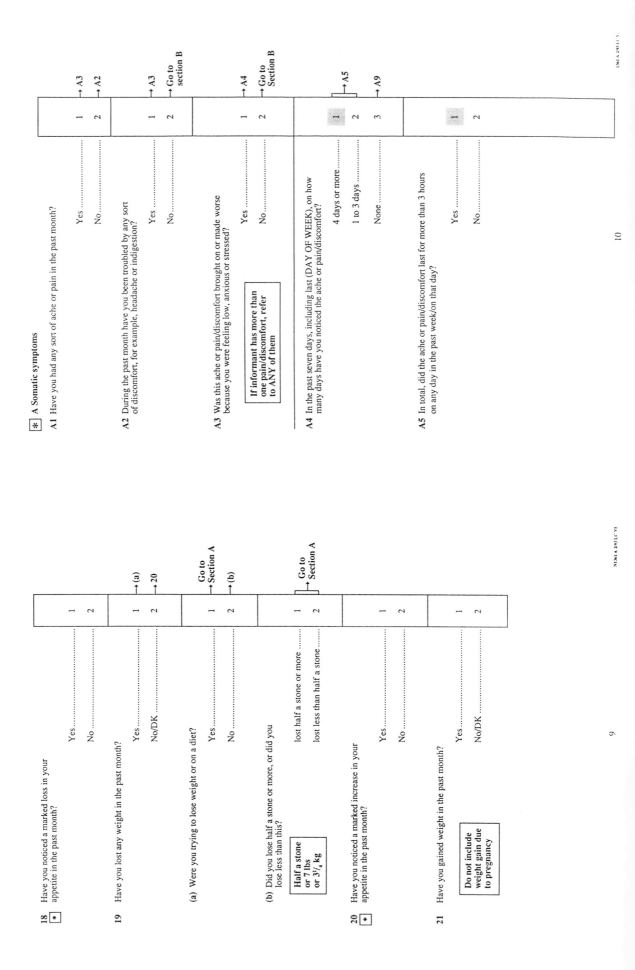

18 [*] Have you noticed a marked loss in your appetite in the past month?

Yes 1
No 2

19 Have you lost any weight in the past month?

Yes .... 1 → (a)
No/DK .... 2 → 20

(a) Were you trying to lose weight or on a diet?

Yes .... 1 → **Go to Section A**
No .... 2 → (b)

(b) Did you lose half a stone or more, or did you lose less than this?

lost half a stone or more ...... 1 → **Go to Section A**
lost less than half a stone 2

[box] **Half a stone or 7 lbs or 3¼ kg**

20 [*] Have you noticed a marked increase in your appetite in the past month?

Yes 1
No 2

21 Have you gained weight in the past month?

Yes 1
No/DK 2

[box] **Do not include weight gain due to pregnancy**

---

[*] A Somatic symptoms

A1 Have you had any sort of ache or pain in the past month?

Yes .... 1 → A3
No .... 2 → A2

A2 During the past month have you been troubled by any sort of discomfort, for example, headache or indigestion?

Yes .... 1 → A3
No .... 2 → **Go to section B**

A3 Was this ache or pain/discomfort brought on or made worse because you were feeling low, anxious or stressed?

Yes .... 1 → A4
No .... 2 → **Go to Section B**

[box] **If informant has more than one pain/discomfort, refer to ANY of them**

A4 In the past seven days, including last (DAY OF WEEK), on how many days have you noticed the ache or pain/discomfort?

4 days or more .... 1 ┐
1 to 3 days .... 2 ┘→ A5
None .... 3 → A9

A5 In total, did the ache or pain/discomfort last for more than 3 hours on any day in the past week/on that day?

Yes 1
No 2

A6 In the past week, has the ache or pain/discomfort been

Running prompt

very unpleasant	1
a little unpleasant	2
or not unpleasant?	3

A7 Has the ache or pain/discomfort bothered you when you were doing something interesting in the past week?

Yes	1
No/has not done anything interesting	2

A8 How long have you been feeling this ache or pain/discomfort as you have just described?

Show card 2

less than 2 weeks	1
2 weeks but less than 6 months	2
6 months but less than 1 year	3
1 year but less than 2 years	4
2 years or more	5

A9 Interviewer check:

Sum codes which you have ringed in the shaded boxes at A4, A5, A6 and A7.

Ring '0' if sum of codes is zero	0
or	
enter score ——————	

→ Insert score on check card, then go to section B

✳ B Fatigue

B1 Have you noticed that you've been getting tired in the past month?

Yes	1	→ B3
No	2	→ B2

B2 During the past month, have you felt you've been lacking in energy?

Yes	1	→ B3
No	2	→ Go to section C

B3 Do you know why you have been feeling tired/lacking in energy?

Yes	1	→ (a)
No	2	→ B4

(a) What is the main reason? Can you choose from this card?

Show card 3

Code one only

Problems with sleep	1	
Medication	2	
Physical illness	3	→ B4
Working too hard (inc. housework, looking after baby)	4	
Stress, worry or other psychological reason	5	
Physical exercise	6	→ Go to section C
Other	7	→ B4

B4 In the past seven days, including last (DAY OF WEEK) on how many days have you felt tired/lacking in energy?

4 days or more	1	→ B5
1 to 3 days	2	
None	3	→ B10

B5 Have you felt tired/lacking in energy for more than 3 hours in total on any day in the past week?

Exclude time spent sleeping

Yes	1
No	2

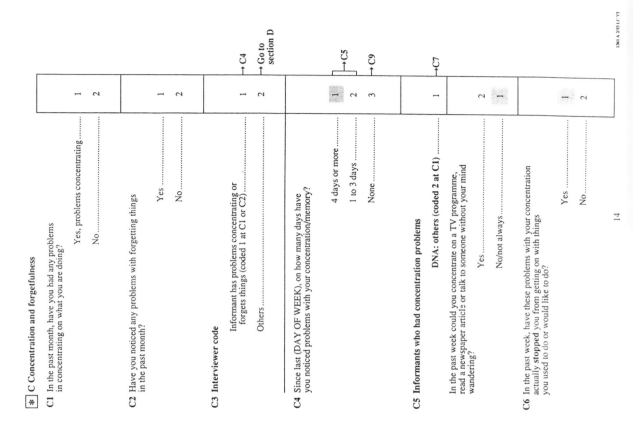

* C Concentration and forgetfulness

C1 In the past month, have you had any problems in concentrating on what you are doing?

Yes, problems concentrating 1
No 2

C2 Have you noticed any problems with forgetting things in the past month?

Yes 1
No 2

C3 Interviewer code

Informant has problems concentrating or forgets things (coded 1 at C1 or C2) ...... 1 → C4
Others ...... 2 → Go to section D

C4 Since last (DAY OF WEEK), on how many days have you noticed problems with your concentration/memory?

4 days or more ...... 1 ┐→ C5
1 to 3 days ...... 2 ┘
None ...... 3 → C9

C5 Informants who had concentration problems

DNA: others (coded 2 at C1) ...... 1 → C7

In the past week could you concentrate on a TV programme, read a newspaper article or talk to someone without your mind wandering?

Yes 2
No/not always 1

C6 In the past week, have these problems with your concentration actually **stopped** you from getting on with things you used to do or would like to do?

Yes 1
No 2

14

B6 Have you felt so tired/lacking in energy that you've had to push yourself to get things done during the past week?

Yes, on at least one occasion 1
No 2

B7 Have you felt tired/lacking in energy when doing things that you enjoy during the past week?

Yes, at least once ...... 1 → B9
No ...... 2 → B8

Spontaneous   Does not enjoy anything 3

B8 Have you in the past week felt tired/lacking in energy when doing things that you **used** to enjoy?

Yes 1
No 2

B9 How long have you been feeling tired/lacking in energy in the way you have just described?

less than 2 weeks 1
2 weeks but less than 6 months 2
6 months but less than 1 year 3
1 year but less than 2 years 4
2 years or more 5

Show card 2

B10 Interviewer check:
Sum codes which you have ringed in the shaded boxes at B4, B5, B6, B7 and B8.

Ring '0' if sum of codes is zero ... 0 → Insert score on check card, then go to section C
or
enter score ———

13

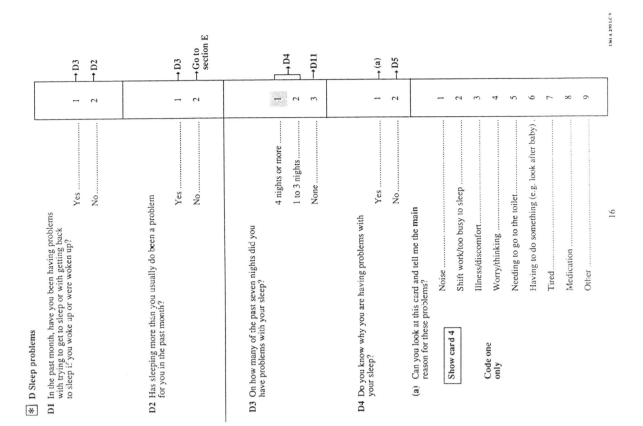

* D Sleep problems

D1 In the past month, have you been having problems with trying to get to sleep or with getting back to sleep if you woke up or were woken up?

Yes .... 1 → D3
No .... 2 → D2

D2 Has sleeping more than you usually do been a problem for you in the past month?

Yes .... 1 → D3
No .... 2 → Go to section E

D3 On how many of the past seven nights did you have problems with your sleep?

4 nights or more .... 1 ⎤
1 to 3 nights .... 2 ⎦ → D4
None .... 3 → D11

D4 Do you know why you are having problems with your sleep?

Yes .... 1 → (a)
No .... 2 → D5

(a) Can you look at this card and tell me the main reason for these problems?

| Show card 4 |

Code one only

Noise 1
Shift work/too busy to sleep 2
Illness/discomfort 3
Worry/thinking 4
Needing to go to the toilet 5
Having to do something (e.g. look after baby) 6
Tired 7
Medication 8
Other 9

1361 A 293 LCV

16

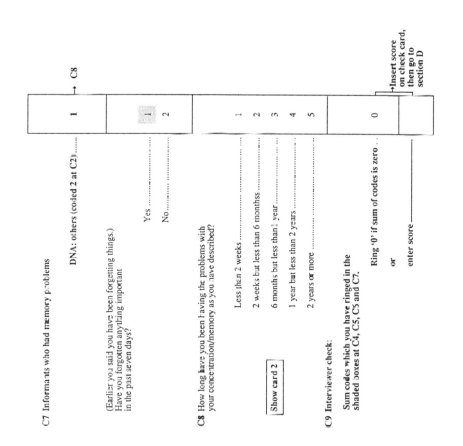

C7 Informants who had memory problems

DNA: others (coded 2 at C2) .... 1 → C8

(Earlier you said you have been forgetting things.) Have you forgotten anything important in the past seven days?

Yes 1
No 2

C8 How long have you been having the problems with your concentration/memory as you have described?

| Show card 2 |

Less than 2 weeks 1
2 weeks but less than 6 months 2
6 months but less than 1 year 3
1 year but less than 2 years 4
2 years or more 5

C9 Interviewer check:

Sum codes which you have ringed in the shaded boxes at C4, C5, C6 and C7.

Ring '0' if sum of codes is zero 0
or
enter score _____ → Insert score on check card, then go to section D

1360 A 293 LCV5

15

D5 Informants who had problems trying to get (back) to sleep

DNA : others (coded 2 at D1) .... 1 → D8

Thinking about the night you had the least sleep in the past week, how long did you spend **trying** to get to sleep? (If you woke up or were woken up I want you to allow a quarter of an hour to get back to sleep).

Only include time spent **trying to get to sleep**.

Less than 1/4 hr .... 3 → **Go to D11 and code '0'**
At least 1/4 hr but less than 1 hr .... 1 → D7
At least 1 hr but less than 3 hrs 2
3 hrs or more .... 2 → D6

D6 In the past week, on how many nights did you spend 3 or more hours trying to get to sleep?

4 nights or more 1
1 to 3 nights 2
None 3

D7 Do you wake more than two hours earlier than you need to and then find you can't get back to sleep?

Yes .... 1 → D10
No 2

D8 Informants who slept more than usual

Thinking about the night you slept the longest in the past week, how much longer did you sleep compared with how long you normally sleep for?

Less than 1/4 hr .... 3 → **Go to D11 and code '0'**
At least 1/4 hr but less than 1 hr .... 1 → D10
At least 1 hr but less than 3 hrs 2
3 hrs or more .... 2 → D9

D9 In the past week, on how many nights did you sleep for more than 3 hours longer than you usually do?

4 nights or more 1
1 to 3 nights 2
None 3

17

D10 How long have you had these problems with your sleep as you have described?

Show card 2

less than 2 weeks 1
2 weeks but less than 6 months 2
6 months but less than 1 year 3
1 year but less than 2 years 4
2 years or more 5

D11 Interviewer check:

Sum codes which you have ringed in the shaded boxes at D3, D5, D6, D8 and D9.

Ring '0' if sum of codes is zero (or if coded 3 at D5 or D8) 0

or

enter score → Insert score on Check card, then go to section E

18

E Irritability

E1 Many people become irritable or short tempered at times, though they may not show it.

Have you felt irritable or short tempered with those around you in the past month?

Yes/no more than usual	1	→ E3
No	2	→ E2

E2 During the past month did you get short tempered or angry over things which now seem trivial when you look back on them?

Yes	1	→ E3
No	2	→ Go to section F

E3 Since last (DAY OF WEEK), on how many days have you felt irritable or short tempered/angry?

4 days or more	1	→ E4
1 to 3 days	2	
None	3	→ E11

E4 What sort of things made you irritable or short tempered/angry in the past week?

E5 In total, have you felt irritable or short tempered/angry for more than one hour (on any day in the past week)?

Yes	1
No	2

E6 During the past week, have you felt so irritable or short tempered/angry that you have wanted to shout at someone, even if you haven't actually shouted?

Yes	1
No	2

19

E7 In the past seven days, have you had arguments, rows or quarrels or lost your temper with anyone?

Yes	1	→ (a)
No	2	→ E10

(a) Did this happen once or more than once (in the past week)?

Once	1	→ E8
More than once	2	→ E9

E8 Do you think this was justified?

Yes, justified	2	
No, not justified	1	→ E10

E9 Do you think this was justified on every occasion?

Yes	2	
No, at least one was unjustified	1	→ E10

E10 How long have you been feeling irritable or short tempered/angry as you have described?

Show card 2

less than 2 weeks	1
two weeks but less than 6 months	2
6 months but less than 1 year	3
1 year but less than 2 years	4
2 years or more	5

E11 Interviewer check:

Sum codes which you have ringed in the shaded boxes at E3, E5, E6, E8 and E9.

Ring '0' if sum of codes is zero	0	→ Insert score on Check card, then go to section F
or		
enter score		

20

115

✱ F Worry about physical health

F1 Many people get concerned about their physical health. In the past month, have you been at all worried about your physical health?

> Include women who are worried about their pregnancy

Yes, worried .... 1 → F3
No/concerned .... 2 → F2

F2 Informants who have no problems with physical health

DNA : has a physical health problem shown at 11a page 6 .... 1 → Go to section G

During the past month, did you find yourself worrying that you might have a serious physical illness?

Yes .... 1 → F3
No .... 2 → Go to section G

F3 Thinking about the past seven days, including last (DAY OF WEEK), on how many days have you found yourself worrying about your physical health/that you might have a serious physical illness?

4 days or more .... 1 ⎤→ F4
1 to 3 days .... 2 ⎦
None .... 3 → F8

F4 In your opinion, have you been worrying too much in view of your actual health?

Yes 1
No 2

F5 In the past week, has this worrying been

Running prompt

very unpleasant 1
a little unpleasant 2
or not unpleasant? 3

21

F6 In the past week, have you been able to take your mind off your health worries at least once, by doing something else?

Yes 2
No, could not be distracted once 1

F7 How long have you been worrying about your physical health in the way you have described?

Show card 2

less than 2 weeks 1
2 weeks but less than 6 months 2
6 months but less than 1 year 3
1 year but less than 2 years 4
2 years or more 5

F8 Interviewer check:

Sum codes which you have ringed in the shaded boxes at F3, F4, F5 and F6.

Ring '0' if sum of codes is zero 0

or

enter score ──────► Insert score on Check card, then go to section G

22

G Depression

G1 Almost everyone becomes sad, miserable or depressed at times.
Have you had a spell of feeling sad, miserable or depressed in the past month?

Yes 1
No 2

G2 During the past month, have you been able to enjoy or take an interest in things as much as you usually do?

Yes 1
No/no enjoyment or interest 2

G3 Interviewer check:

Code first that applies

Informant felt sad, miserable or depressed (coded 1 at G1) .... 1 →**G4**
Informant unable to enjoy or take an interest (coded 2 at G2) .... 2 →**G5**
Others .... 3 →**Go to Section I, page 28**

G4 In the past week have you had a spell of feeling sad, miserable or depressed?

Use informant's own words if possible

Yes 1
No .... 2 →**See G5**

G5 Informants who were unable to enjoy or take an interest in things

DNA: coded 1 at G2 .... 1 →**See G6**

In the past week, have you been able to enjoy or take an interest in things as much as usual?

Use informant's own words if possible

Yes 1
No/no enjoyment or interest 2

G6 Informants who felt sad, miserable or depressed or unable to enjoy or take an interest in things in the past week (coded 1 at G4 or G5)

DNA: others .... 1 →**Go to G11**

Since last (DAY OF WEEK) on how many days have you felt sad, miserable or depressed/unable to enjoy or take an interest in things?

4 days or more 1
2 to 3 days 2
1 day 3

G7 Have you felt sad, miserable or depressed/unable to enjoy or take an interest in things for more than 3 hours in total (on any day in the past week)?

Yes 1
No 2

G8 (a) What sorts of things made you feel sad, miserable or depressed/unable to enjoy or take an interest in things in the past week? Can you choose from this card?

Ring code(s) in column (a).

Show card 5

	(a) Code all that apply	(b) Code one only
Members of the family	01	01
Relationship with spouse/partner	02	02
Relationships with friends	03	03
Housing	04	04
Money/bills	05	05
Own physical health (inc. pregnancy)	06	06
Own mental health	07	07
Work or lack of work (inc. student)	08	08
Legal difficulties	09	09
Political issues/the news	10	10
Other	11	11
Don't know/no main thing	99	99

(b) DNA : Only one item coded at (a) .... 1 →**G9**

What was the main thing?
Ring code in column (b)

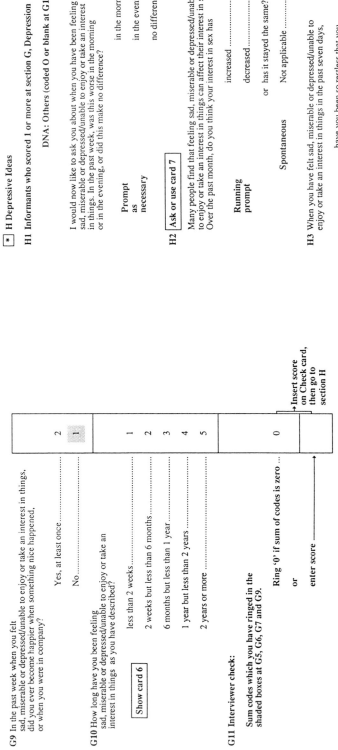

G9 In the past week when you felt sad, miserable or depressed/unable to enjoy or take an interest in things, did you ever become happier when something nice happened, or when you were in company?

Yes, at least once ... 2
No ... 1

G10 How long have you been feeling sad, miserable or depressed/unable to enjoy or take an interest in things as you have described?

Show card 6

less than 2 weeks ... 1
2 weeks but less than 6 months ... 2
6 months but less than 1 year ... 3
1 year but less than 2 years ... 4
2 years or more ... 5

G11 Interviewer check:

Sum codes which you have ringed in the shaded boxes at G5, G6, G7 and G9.

Ring '0' if sum of codes is zero ... 0
or
enter score ...

→ Insert score on Check card, then go to section H

25

* H Depressive Ideas

H1 Informants who scored 1 or more at section G, Depression ... 1 → Go to section I

DNA: Others (coded O or blank at G11)

I would now like to ask you about when you have been feeling sad, miserable or depressed/unable to enjoy or take an interest in things. In the past week, was this worse in the morning or in the evening, or did this make no difference?

Prompt as necessary
in the morning ... 1
in the evening ... 2
no difference/other ... 3

H2 Ask or use card 7

Many people find that feeling sad, miserable or depressed/unable to enjoy or take an interest in things can affect their interest in sex. Over the past month, do you think your interest in sex has

Running prompt
increased ... 1
decreased ... 2
or has it stayed the same? ... 3

Spontaneous Not applicable ... 4

H3 When you have felt sad, miserable or depressed/unable to enjoy or take an interest in things in the past seven days,

	Yes	No
have you been so restless that you couldn't sit still?	1	2
Individual prompt: have you been doing things more slowly, for example, walking more slowly?	1	2
have you been less talkative than normal?	1	2

H4 Now, thinking about the past seven days have you on at least one occasion felt guilty or blamed yourself when things went wrong when it hasn't been your fault?

Yes, at least once ... 1
No ... 2

H5 During the past week, have you been feeling you are not as good as other people?

Yes ... 1
No ... 2

H6 Have you felt hopeless at all during the past seven days, for instance about your future?

Yes ... 1
No ... 2

26

Page 27

H7 Interviewer check

Informant felt guilty, not as good as others or hopeless (coded 1 at H4 or H5 or H6)	1	→ H8
Others (coded 2 at H4, H5 and H6)	2	→ read H10

H8 Ask or use card 8

In the past week have you felt that life isn't worth living?

Yes	1	→ H9
Spontaneous: Yes, but not in the past week	2	
No	3	→ read H10

H9 Ask or use card 9

In the past week, have you thought of killing yourself?

Yes	1	→ (a)
Spontaneous: Yes, but not in the past week	2	
No	3	→ read H10

(a) Have you talked to your doctor about these thoughts (of killing yourself)?

Yes	1	→ read H10
Spontaneous: No, but has talked to other people	2	→ read (b)
No	3	

(b) (You have said that you are thinking about committing suicide)

Since this is a very serious matter it is important that you talk to your doctor about these thoughts. → read H10

H10 Thank you for answering those questions on how you have been feeling. I would now like to ask you a few questions about worrying.)

H11 Interviewer check:

Sum codes which you have ringed in the shaded boxes at H4, H5, H6, H8 and H9.

Ring '0' if sum of codes is zero	0	Insert score on Check card, then go to section I
or		
enter score _____		

Maximum score on this section is 5

27

Page 28

* I Worry

I1 (The next few questions are about worrying.)
In the past month, did you find yourself worrying more than you needed to about things?

Yes, worrying	1	→ I3
No/concerned	2	→ I2

I2 Have you had any worries at all in the past month?

Yes	1	→ I3
No	2	→ Go to section J

I3 (a) Can you look at this card and tell me what sorts of things you worried about in the past month?

Ring code(s) in column (a).

	(a) Code all that apply	(b) Code one only
Members of the family	01	01
Relationship with spouse/partner	02	02
Relationships with friends	03	03
Housing	04	04
Money/bills	05	05
Own physical health (inc. pregnancy)	06	06
Own mental health	07	07
Work or lack of work (inc student)	08	08
Legal difficulties	09	09
Political issues/the news	10	10
Other	11	11
Don't know/no main thing	99	99

Show card 10

DNA : Only one item coded at (a) ... 1 → I4

(b) What was the main thing you worried about?
Ring code in column (b).

I4 Interviewer check:

Informant worries about physical health (coded 06 at I3(a))	1	See instruction below, then go to I5
Others (not coded 06 at I3(a))	2	→ I6

Make a note on Check flap to go to section F to record this worry about physical health, if not already recorded.

28

119

I 5 Interviewer check:

Informant is **only** worried about physical health
(only code 06 is rung at I3(a)) .... 1 → **Go to section J**

Informant had other worries (I3(a) is multi-coded) .... 2 → **read (a)**

(a) For the next few questions, I want you to think about the worries you have had **other** than those about your physical health.

I 6 On how many of the past seven days have you been worrying about things (other than your physical health)?

4 days or more .... 1 → **I7**

1 to 3 days 2

None .... 3 → **I11**

I 7 In your opinion, have you been worrying too much in view of your circumstances?

Yes 1

No 2

> Refer to worries other than those about physical health

I 8 In the past week, has this worrying been:

Running prompt

very unpleasant 1

a little unpleasant 2

or not unpleasant? 3

> Refer to worries other than those about physical health

I 9 Have you worried for more than 3 hours in total on any one of the past seven days?

Yes 1

No 2

> Refer to worries other than those about physical health

I 10 How long have you been worrying about things in the way that you have described?

Show card I1

less than 2 weeks 1

2 weeks but less than 6 months 2

6 months but less than 1 year 3

1 year but less than 2 years 4

2 years or more 5

I 11 Interviewer check:

Sum codes which you have ringed in the shaded boxes at I6, I7, I8 and I9.

Ring '0' if sum of codes is zero ... 0

or

enter score .... → **Insert score on Check card, then go to section J**

J Anxiety

J1 Have you been feeling anxious or nervous in the past month?

Yes, anxious or nervous	1	→ J3
No	2	→ J2

J2 In the past month, did you ever find your muscles felt tense or that you couldn't relax?

Yes	1
No	2

J3 Some people have phobias; they get nervous or uncomfortable about specific things or situations when there is no real danger. For instance they may get nervous when speaking or eating in front of strangers, when they are far from home or in crowded rooms, or they may have a fear of heights. Others become nervous at the sight of things like blood or spiders.

In the past month have you felt anxious, nervous or tense about any specific things or situations when there was no real danger?

Yes	1
No	2

J4 Interviewer check:

Informant reports anxiety and also a phobia (coded 1 at J1 or J2, and coded 1 at J3)	1	→ J5
Informant reports only general anxiety (coded 1 at J1 or J2, and coded 2 at J3)	2	→ J7
Others	3	→ Go to section K

J5 In the past month, when you felt anxious/nervous/tense, was this always brought on by the phobia about some specific situation or thing or did you sometimes feel generally anxious/nervous/tense?

Always brought on by phobia	1	→ Go to section K
Sometimes felt generally anxious	2	→ J6

J6 The next questions are concerned with **general anxiety/nervousness/tension only**.
I will ask you about the anxiety which is brought on by the phobia about specific things or situations later.

On how many of the past seven days have you felt **generally anxious/nervous/tense**?

4 days or more	1	→ J8
1 to 3 days	2	→ J8
None	3	→ J12

J7 On how many of the past seven days have you felt generally anxious/nervous/tense?

4 days or more	1	→ J8
1 to 3 days	2	→ J8
None	3	→ J12

J8 In the past week, has your anxiety/nervousness/tension been:

Running prompt

very unpleasant	1
a little unpleasant	2
or not unpleasant?	3

J9 In the past week, when you've been anxious/nervous/tense, have you had any of the symptoms shown on this card?

Show card 12

Yes	1	→ (a)
No	2	→ J10

(a) Which of these symptoms did you have when you felt anxious/nervous/tense?

Code all that apply

Heart racing or pounding	1
Hands sweating or shaking	2
Feeling dizzy	3
Difficulty getting your breath	4
Butterflies in stomach	5
Dry mouth	6
Nausea or feeling as though you wanted to vomit	7

If informant had any of **these symptoms**, check J9 is coded 1, '**Yes**'.

J10 Have you felt anxious/nervous/tense for more than 3 hours in total on any one of the past seven days?

Yes 1
No 2

J11 How long have you had these feelings of general anxiety/nervousness/tension as you described?

Show card 11

less than 2 weeks 1
2 weeks but less than 6 months 2
6 months but less than 1 year 3
1 year but less than 2 years 4
2 years or more 5

J12 Interviewer check:

Sum codes which you have ringed in the shaded boxes at J6, J7, J8, J9 and J10.

Ring '0' if sum of codes is zero 0

or

enter score .... → Insert score on Check card, then go to section K

---

* **K Phobias**

K1 Interviewer check:

Informants who had phobic anxiety in the past month (coded 1 at J3) .... 1 → K3(a)
Others .... 2 → K2

K2 Sometimes people avoid a specific situation or thing because the have a phobia about it. For instance, some people avoid eating in public or avoid going to busy places because it would make them feel nervous or anxious.

In the past month, have you avoided any situation or thing because it would have made you feel nervous or anxious, even though there was no real danger?

Yes .... 1 → K3(b)
No .... 2 → See section L

K3(a) Can you look at this card and tell me which of the situations or things listed made you the **most** anxious/nervous/tense in the past month? Ring code at (b), then go to K4

Show card 13

(b) Can you look at this card and tell me, which of these situations or things did you avoid the **most** in the past month?

Show card 13

Code one only

Crowds or public places, including travelling alone or being far from home 1
Enclosed spaces 2
Social situations, including eating or speaking in public, being watched or stared at 3
The sight of blood or injury 4
Any specific single cause including insects, spiders and heights 5
Other (specify) 6

K4 Informants who had phobic anxiety in past month .... 1 → K7

DNA: others (coded 2 at K1) .... 1 → K5

In the past seven days, how many times have you felt nervous or anxious about (SITUATION/THING)?

4 times or more .... 1 → K5
1 to 3 times 2
None .... 3 → K6

33

34

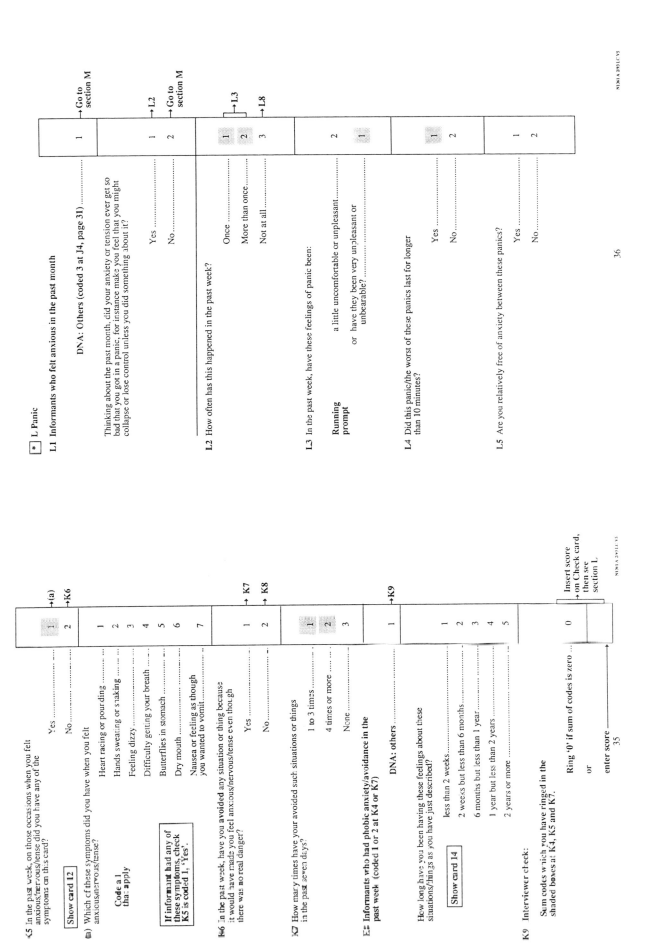

K5 In the past week, on those occasions when you felt anxious/nervous/tense did you have any of the symptoms on this card?

Yes ... 1 → (a)
No ... 2 → K6

Show card 12

(a) Which of these symptoms did you have when you felt anxious/nervous/tense?

Code all that apply

Heart racing or pounding ... 1
Hands sweating or shaking ... 2
Feeling dizzy ... 3
Difficulty getting your breath ... 4
Butterflies in stomach ... 5
Dry mouth ... 6
Nausea or feeling as though you wanted to vomit ... 7

If informant had any of these symptoms, check K5 is coded 1, 'Yes'.

K6 In the past week, have you avoided any situation or thing because it would have made you feel anxious/nervous/tense even though there was no real danger?

Yes ... 1 → K7
No ... 2 → K8

K7 How many times have your avoided such situations or things in the past seven days?

1 to 3 times ... 1
4 times or more ... 2 → K9
None ... 3

K8 Informants who had phobic anxiety/avoidance in the past week (coded 1 or 2 at K4 or K7)

DNA: others ... 1 → K9

How long have you been having these feelings about these situations/things as you have just described?

Show card 14

less than 2 weeks ... 1
2 weeks but less than 6 months ... 2
6 months but less than 1 year ... 3
1 year but less than 2 years ... 4
2 years or more ... 5

K9 Interviewer check:

Sum codes which you have ringed in the shaded boxes at K4, K5 and K7.

Ring '0' if sum of codes is zero ... 0
or
enter score

Insert score on Check card, then see section L

35

---

* L Panic

L1 Informants who felt anxious in the past month

DNA: Others (coded 3 at J4, page 31) ... 1 → Go to section M

Thinking about the past month, did your anxiety or tension ever get so bad that you got in a panic, for instance make you feel that you might collapse or lose control unless you did something about it?

Yes ... 1 → L2
No ... 2 → Go to section M

L2 How often has this happened in the past week?

Once ... 1
More than once ... 2 → L3
Not at all ... 3 → L8

L3 In the past week, have these feelings of panic been:

Running prompt   a little uncomfortable or unpleasant ... 2
or have they been very unpleasant or unbearable? ... 1

L4 Did this panic/the worst of these panics last for longer than 10 minutes?

Yes ... 1
No ... 2

L5 Are you relatively free of anxiety between these panics?

Yes ... 1
No ... 2

36

L6 Informants who had phobic anxiety

DNA: Others (coded 2 at K1) .... | 1 → L7

Refer to situation/thing at K3.

Is this panic always brought on by (SITUATION/THING)?

Yes .... | 1
No .... | 2

L7 How long have you been having these feelings of panic as you have described?

| Show card 14 |

less than 2 weeks .... | 1
2 weeks but less than 6 months .... | 2
6 months but less than 1 year .... | 3
1 year but less than 2 years .... | 4
2 years or more .... | 5

L8 Interviewer check:

Sum codes which you have ringed in the shaded boxes at L2, L3, and L4.

Ring '0' if sum of codes is zero ... | 0 → **Insert score on Check card, then go to section M**

or

enter score →

※ M Compulsions

M1 In the past month, did you find that you kept on doing things over and over again when you knew you had already done them, for instance checking things like taps or washing yourself when you had already done so?

Yes .... | 1 → M2
No .... | 2 → Go to section N

M2 On how many days in the past week did you find yourself doing things over again that you had already done?

4 days or more .... | 1 ┐
1 to 3 days .... | 2 ┘ → M3
None .... | 3 → M9

M3 Since last (DAY OF WEEK) what sorts of things have you done over and over again?

M4 During the past week, have you tried to stop yourself repeating (BEHAVIOUR)/doing any of these things over again?

Yes .... | 1
No .... | 2

M5 Has repeating (BEHAVIOUR)/doing any of these things over again made you upset or annoyed with yourself in the past week?

Yes, upset or annoyed .... | 1
No, not at all .... | 2

124

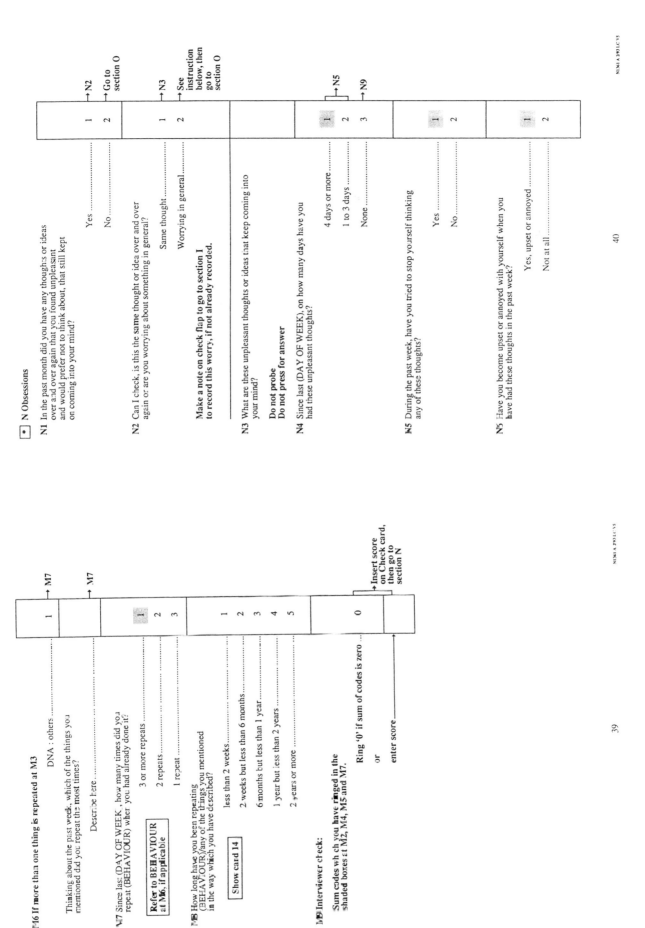

M6 If more than one thing is repeated at M3

DNA : others .... 1 → M7

Thinking about the past week, which of the things you mentioned did you repeat the most times?

Describe here .... → M7

M7 Since last (DAY OF WEEK), how many times did you repeat (BEHAVIOUR) when you had already done it?

Refer to **BEHAVIOUR** at **M6**, if applicable

3 or more repeats 1
2 repeats 2
1 repeat 3

M8 Show card 14

How long have you been repeating (BEHAVIOUR)/any of the things you mentioned in the way which you have described?

less than 2 weeks 1
2 weeks but less than 6 months 2
6 months but less than 1 year 3
1 year but less than 2 years 4
2 years or more 5

M9 Interviewer check:

Sum codes which you have **ringed** in the shaded boxes at **M2, M4, M5 and M7.**

Ring '0' if sum of codes is zero .... 0 → Insert score on Check card, then go to section N

or

enter score _____

☀ N Obsessions

N1 In the past month did you have any thoughts or ideas over and over again that you found unpleasant and would prefer not to think about, that still kept on coming into your mind?

Yes .... 1 → N2
No .... 2 → Go to section O

N2 Can I check, is this the **same** thought or idea over and over again or are you worrying about something in general?

Same thought .... 1 → N3
Worrying in general .... 2 → See instruction below, then go to section O

Make a note on check flap to go to section I to record this worry, if not already recorded.

N3 What are these unpleasant thoughts or ideas that keep coming into your mind?

Do not probe
Do not press for answer

N4 Since last (DAY OF WEEK), on how many days have you had these unpleasant thoughts?

4 days or more 1
1 to 3 days .... 2 ⌐ → N5
None .... 3 → N9

N5 During the past week, have you tried to stop yourself thinking any of these thoughts?

Yes 1
No 2

N6 Have you become upset or annoyed with yourself when you have had these thoughts in the past week?

Yes, upset or annoyed 1
Not at all 2

39

40

N7 In the past week, was the longest episode of having such thoughts :

Running prompt

a quarter of an hour or longer 1

or was it less than this? 2

N8 How long have you been having these thoughts in the way which you have just described?

| Show card 14 |

less than 2 weeks 1

2 weeks but less than 6 months 2

6 months but less than 1 year 3

1 year but less than 2 years 4

2 years or more 5

N9 **Interviewer check:**

Sum codes which you have ringed in the shaded boxes at N4, N5, N6 and N7.

Ring '0' if sum of codes is zero ... 0

or

enter score →

→ **Insert score on Check card, then go to section O**

41

SA TUGE A 29 TUM N

---

* O Overall effects

Informants who scored 2 or more on any section, A to N.

DNA: Others (All section scores 0 or 1 on check card) .... 1 → **Complete Check card, then go to Section P, page 43**

Now I would like to ask you how all of these things that you have told me about have affected you overall.

In the past week, has the way you have been feeling ever actually **stopped** you from getting on with things you used to do or would like to do?

Yes .... 1 → (a)

No .... 2 → (b)

(a) In the past week, has the way you have been feeling stopped you doing things once or more than once?

Once .... 1 → **Complete Check card, then go to Section P, page 43**

More than once 2

(b) Has the way you have been feeling made things more difficult even though you have got everything done?

Yes .... 1 → **Complete Check card, then go to Section P, page 43**

No 2

42

SA TUGE A 29 TUM N

126

F. PSQ

F1 Over the past year, have there been times when you felt very happy indeed without a break for days on end?

Yes .... 1 →(a)
Unsure .... 2 →P2
No 3

(a) Was there an obvious reason for this?

Yes .... 1 →P2
Unsure 2
No .... 3 →(b)

(b) Did your relatives or friends think it was strange or complain about it?

Yes .... 1 Screen Positive, Go to P6
Unsure 2
No .... 3 →P2

P2 Over the past year, have you ever felt that your thoughts were directly interfered with or controlled by some outside force or person?

Yes .... 1 →(a)
Unsure .... 2 →P3
No 3

(a) Did this come about in a way that many people would find hard to believe, for instance, through telepathy?

Yes .... 1 Screen Positive, Go to P6
Unsure 2
No .... 3 →P3

43

P3 Over the past year, have there been times when you felt that people were against you?

Yes .... 1 →(a)
Unsure .... 2 →P4
No 3

(a) Have there been times when you felt that people were deliberately acting to harm you or your interests?

Yes .... 1 →(b)
Unsure .... 2 →P4
No 3

(b) Have there been times you felt that a group of people was plotting to cause you serious harm or injury?

Yes .... 1 Screen Positive, Go to P6
Unsure 2
No .... 3 →P4

P4 Over the past year, have there been times when you felt that something strange was going on?

Yes .... 1 →(a)
Unsure .... 2 →P5
No 3

(a) Did you feel it was so strange that other people would find it very hard to believe?

Yes .... 1 Screen Positive, Go to P6
Unsure 2
No .... 3 →P5

44

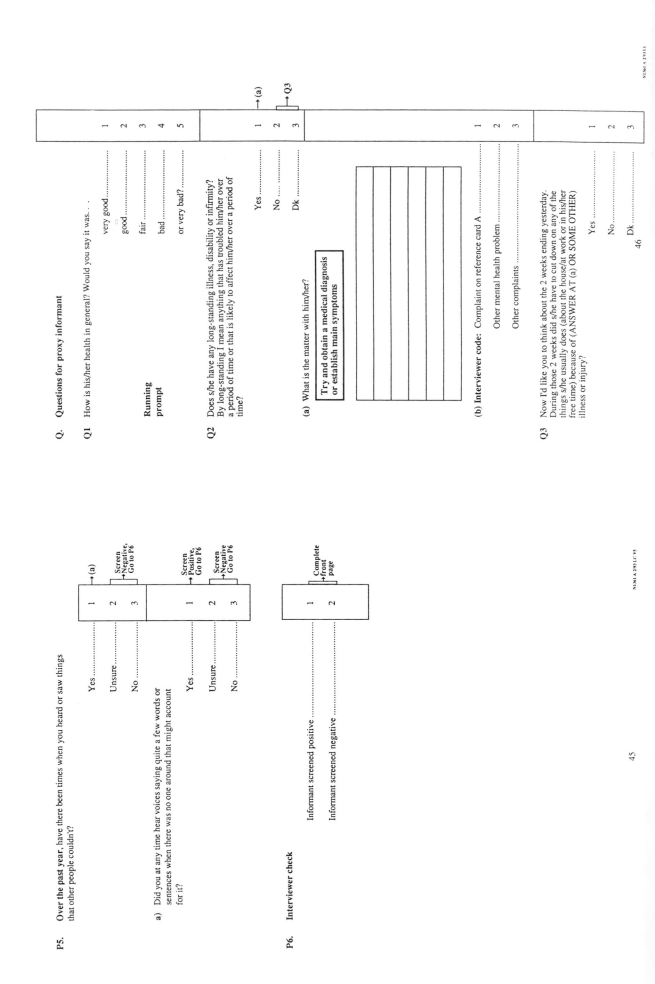

P5. Over the past year, have there been times when you heard or saw things that other people couldn't?

Yes .... 1 → (a)

Unsure .... 2 → Screen Negative, Go to P6

No .... 3 → Screen Negative, Go to P6

a) Did you at any time hear voices saying quite a few words or sentences when there was no one around that might account for it?

Yes .... 1 → Screen Positive, Go to P6

Unsure .... 2 → Screen Negative, Go to P6

No .... 3 → Screen Negative, Go to P6

P6. Interviewer check

Informant screened positive .... 1 → Complete front page

Informant screened negative 2

Q. Questions for proxy informant

Q1 How is his/her health in general? Would you say it was. . .

very good 1

good 2

fair 3

bad 4

or very bad? 5

Running prompt

Q2 Does s/he have any long-standing illness, disability or infirmity? By long-standing I mean anything that has troubled him/her over a period of time or that is likely to affect him/her over a period of time?

Yes .... 1 → (a)

No .... 2 → Q3

Dk .... 3 → Q3

(a) What is the matter with him/her?

Try and obtain a medical diagnosis or establish main symptoms

(b) Interviewer code: Complaint on reference card A 1

Other mental health problem 2

Other complaints 3

Q3 Now I'd like you to think about the 2 weeks ending yesterday. During those 2 weeks did s/he have to cut down on any of the things s/he usually does (about the house/at work or in his/her free time) because of (ANSWER AT (a) OR SOME OTHER) illness or injury?

Yes 1

No 2

Dk 3

46

45

Q6 During the two weeks ending yesterday, apart from any visit to a hospital, did s/he talk to a doctor for any reason at all, either in person or by telephone?

Yes .... 1 → (a)
No 2
Dk .... 3 → Q7

Exclude: consultations made on behalf of children under 16 and persons outside the household

(a) How many times did s/he talk to a doctor in these two weeks?

Enter number — [Dk = 99]

Q7 In the past twelve months, has s/he spoken to a GP or family doctor on his/her own behalf, either in person or by telephone about a physical illness or complaint?

Yes 1
No 2
Dk 3

Q8 In the past twelve months has s/he spoken to a GP or family doctor on his/her own behalf, either in person or by telephone about being anxious or depressed or a mental, nervous or emotional problem?

Yes .... 1 → (a)
No .... 2 → Go to front page
Dk 3

(a) What did the doctor say was the matter with him/her.

Try and obtain a medical diagnosis or establish main symptoms

(b) Interviewer code: Complaint on reference card A 1
Other mental health problem .... 2 → Go to front page
Other complaints 3

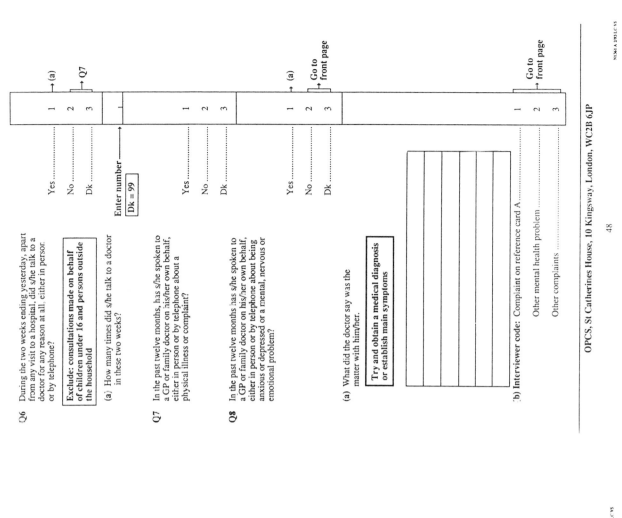

OPCS, St Catherines House, 10 Kingsway, London, WC2B 6JP

48

N3M1A 2931LC Y5

Q4 (May I just check), is s/he taking any pills or tablets or any other medicine by mouth which have been prescribed for him/her?

Yes .... 1 → (a)
No 2
Dk .... 3 → Q5

(a) What is the name of the pills, tablets or medicine s/he is taking?

Ask to look at bottle or box if clarification is required

(b) Interviewer code: Medication on reference card B 1
Other 2

Q5 Is s/he getting a regular course of injections?

Yes .... 1 → (a)
No 2
Dk .... 3 → Q6

(a) What is it? (What are they?)

(b) Interviewer code: Injection on reference card B 1
Other 2

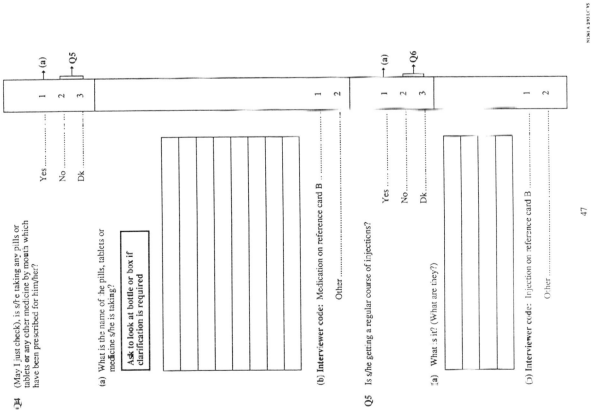

47

N3M1A 2931LC Y5

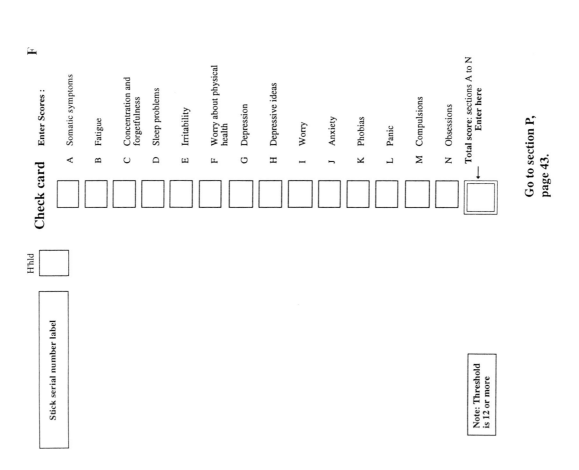

F

Check card   Enter Scores :

A   Somatic symptoms

B   Fatigue

C   Concentration and forgetfulness

D   Sleep problems

E   Irritability

F   Worry about physical health

G   Depression

H   Depressive ideas

I   Worry

J   Anxiety

K   Phobias

L   Panic

M   Compulsions

N   Obsessions

Total score: sections A to N
Enter here

Go to section P, page 43.

H'hld

Stick serial number label

Note: Threshold is 12 or more

Reference Card A

- Auditory hallucinations
- Bipolar affective disorder
- Catatonic schizophrenia
- Chronic schizophrenia
- Hallucinations
- Hearing voices
- Hebephrenic schizophrenia
- Hypomania
- Mania
- Manic depression
- Manic depressive psychosis
- Mental illness
- Mentally disturbed
- Mild psychosis
- Mild schizophrenia
- Mood swings
- Neuroleptic
- Paranoia
- Paranoid schizophrenia
- Psychosis
- Psychotic related disorder
- Psychotic tendencies
- Schizo-affective disorder
- Schizophrenia
- Schizophrenic affective disorder
- Simple schizophrenia
- Voices

Reference card B

Anquil	Haldol decanoate
Benperidol	Halperidol
Camcolit	Largactil
Chlorpromazine	Liskonum
Clopixol acuphase	Litarex
Clopixol	Lithium
Clozapine	Loxapac
Clozaril	Loxapine
Depixol	Melleril
Dolmatil	Methotrimeprazine
Dozic	Modecate
Droleptan	Moditen
Droperidol	Moditen ethanate
Fentazin	Neulactil
Fluanxol	Nozinan
Flupenthixol	Orap
Flupenthixol decanoate	Oxypertine
Fluphenazine hydrochloride	Pericyazine
Fluphenazine decanoate	Perphenazine
Fluphenazine enanthate	Phasal
Fluspirilene	Pimozide
Fortunan	Piportil
Haldol	Pipothiazine palmiate

Priadel
Prochloperazine
Promazine hydrochloride
Redeptin
Remoxipride
Roxiam
Serenace
Sparine
Stelazine
Sulphiride
Sulpitl
Thioridazine
Trifluoperazine
Trifluperidol
Zuclopenthixol dihydrochloride
Zuclopenthixol acetate
Zuclopenthixol decanoate

Antipsychotic drugs

Antipsychotic injections

Depot injections

Antimanic drugs

131

N1361   <u>Yellow Schedule</u>   **B**

IN CONFIDENCE

Stick serial number label	H'hld	Date of Interview

Date of Interview: 9 3

(1)

Complete at end of interview.

(i) Type of interview:

Full interview, ... 1
Partial interview ... 2
Refusal ... 3

(ii) Who was interviewed?

Subject ... 1 → **Go to Recall Sheet**
Proxy ... 2 → **(iii) - (iv)**
Both ... 3

(iii) Was subject present during the interview?

Yes - all the time ... 1
Yes - part of the time ... 2
No ... 3

(iv) Reason for proxy:

Subject absent ... 1
Subject incapable due to mental health problems ... 2
Subject too ill ... 3
Subject has speech/hearing problem ... 4
Subject cannot speak English ... 5
Other (specify) ... 6 → **End interview**

Sched. B LC 8393 Y4

1

A   Long-standing illness

A1   Informant has long-standing illness or saw a GP about
a mental, nervous or emotional problem
DNA:Informants coded 2 at qn.11, page 6 <u>and</u> qn.17,
page 8, Schedule A
Proxy informants coded 2 or 3 at Q2, page 46
<u>and</u> Q8, page 48, Schedule A ....

1 → Go to Section B
page 4

Refer to complaints in Schedule A:
For informants, see qn.11a, page 6 <u>and</u> qn.17a, page 8;
For proxy informants, see Q2a, page 46 <u>and</u> Q8a, page 48.

Earlier you told me about (COMPLAINT(s)).
I'd now like to ask you a few more questions about this.

Transcribe details of complaint(s) from Schedule A.

COMPLAINT No. →	1		2		3		4	

(a) Name of complaint
or
Describe main symptoms

Try and obtain
medical diagnosis

(b) How old were you
when your
(COMPLAINT)
started?

Enter AGE →

Code 00 if from birth
Code 99 if DK

(c) For how long has your
(COMPLAINT) been
at its present level?

Enter no. of years →
OR if less than 1 year
Enter no. of months →
(less than 1 month = 00)

(d) In the past week, did
your (COMPLAINT)
actually stop you from
getting on with the
things you usually
do or would like
do?

Yes   1
No   2

5		6		7		8	

Sched. B LC 8993 V4

B. Medication and treatment

B1 DNA: No oral medication or injections (coded 2 at qns.13 and 14, page 7 or if proxy, coded 2 or 3 at Q4 and Q5, page 47, Schedule A)................ [1] → B2

Ring column number when appropriate →

	1	2	3	4	5	6	7	8

(a) Transcribe list of pills, medication or injections from questions 13(a) and 14(a), page 7, or Q4(a) and Q5(a), page 47, Schedule A

   Try and establish brand name. If necessary, ask informant to look at name on bottle or box

   Injection: Ring → [1]

(b) What is it's/their strength?

   If strength of pills not known, describe colour and note what is written on tablet

(c) How many/much are you supposed to have each day?

   Enter number of pills/mls/injections per day →

   OR if less than 1 one a day

   Enter number of pills/mls/injections per month →

   (Less than one per month = 00)

   OFF USE

Spontaneous: Take as needed................ [1]

(d) For what condition do you take them?

   Obtain medical diagnosis AND describe main symptoms

(e) How long have you been having this medication?

   Enter number of years

   OR if less than 1 year

   Enter number of months (Less than 1 month = 0 0)

   OFF USE

Ring column number when appropriate→	1	2	3	4	5	6	7	8
(f) Do you sometimes not take your medication even though you should?								
Yes..........	1 → (g)	1 → (g)	1 → (g)	1 → (g)	1 → (g)	1 → (g)	1 → (g)	1 → (g)
No..........	2 → (i)	2 → (i)	2 → (i)	2 → (i)	2 → (i)	2 → (i)	2 → (i)	2 → (i)
(g) When was the last time this happened?								
Less than 1 week ago	1	1	1	1	1	1	1	1
At least 1 week but less than 1 month ago	2	2	2	2	2	2	2	2
At least 1 month ago	3	3	3	3	3	3	3	3
(h) What was the reason for this? **Code all that apply**								
Forgot.......	1	1	1	1	1	1	1	1
Didn't need it.......	2	2	2	2	2	2	2	2
Don't like to take drugs..	3	3	3	3	3	3	3	3
Side effects.......	4	4	4	4	4	4	4	4
Other.......	5	5	5	5	5	5	5	5
(i) Do you sometimes take more medication/pills than the stated dose?								
Yes..........	1 → (j)	1 → (j)	1 → (j)	1 → (j)	1 → (j)	1 → (j)	1 → (j)	1 → (j)
No..........	2 → (l)	2 → (l)	2 → (l)	2 → (l)	2 → (l)	2 → (l)	2 → (l)	2 → (l)
(j) When was the last time this happened?								
Less than 1 week ago	1	1	1	1	1	1	1	1
At least 1 week but less than 1 month ago	2	2	2	2	2	2	2	2
At least 1 month ago	3	3	3	3	3	3	3	3
(k) What was the reason for this? **Code all that apply**								
Needed more to control symptoms....	1	1	1	1	1	1	1	1
Deliberate overdose.......	2	2	2	2	2	2	2	2
Other.......	3	3	3	3	3	3	3	3

Sched B LC 0399 V4

	1	2	3	4	5	6	7	8
Ring column number when appropriate →								
(l) Transcribe condition from (d), pages 4 and 5.....								
(m) DNA: already asked about this condition in a previous column	X	1 → col 3 or B2	1 → col 4 or B2	1 → col 5 or B2	1 → col 6 or B2	1 → col 7 or B2	1 → col 8 or B2	1 → B2
Have you had any other medication or treatment for (CONDITION AT (l)) which you don't have now — Yes	1 → (n)	1 → (n)	1 → (n)	1 → (n)	1 → (n)	1 → (n)	1 → (n)	1 → (n)
No	2 → (p)	2 → (p)	2 → (p)	2 → (p)	2 → (p)	2 → (p)	2 → (p)	2 → (p)
(n) Did you stop this treatment on your own accord or on professional advice? — Own accord	1 → (o)	1 → (o)	1 → (o)	1 → (o)	1 → (o)	1 → (o)	1 → (o)	1 → (o)
Professional advice	2 → (p)	2 → (p)	2 → (p)	2 → (p)	2 → (p)	2 → (p)	2 → (p)	2 → (p)
⊡ (o) What made you decide to stop this treatment? Code all that apply — Did not work/were not strong enough	1	1	1	1	1	1	1	1
Side effects	2	2	2	2	2	2	2	2
Other	3	3	3	3	3	3	3	3
(p) Have you ever been offered any other medication or treatment for (CONDITION) which you refused? — Yes	1 → (q)	1 → (q)	1 → (q)	1 → (q)	1 → (q)	1 → (q)	1 → (q)	1 → (q)
No	2 → col 2 or B2	2 → col 3 or B2	2 → col 4 or B2	2 → col 5 or B2	2 → col 6 or B2	2 → col 7 or B2	2 → col 8 or B2	2 → B2
(q) What was it?								
	OFF USE	OFF USE	OFF USE	OFF USE	OFF USE	OFF USE	OFF USE	OFF USE
⊡ (r) Why did you refuse it? Code all that apply — Worry about side effects	1	1	1	1	1	1	1	1
Don't like medication/treatment	2	2	2	2	2	2	2	2
Other	3	3	3	3	3	3	3	3

Select BLC 8393 V4

B2 At the moment are you having any counselling or therapy either at home, at a doctor's surgery, a health centre, hospital or clinic?

Yes..... 1 →(a)
No..... 2 → Section C page 12

Ring column no. when appropriate →

	1	2	3
(a) What type of counselling or therapy are you having at the moment?	OFF USE	OFF USE	OFF USE
(b) How often do you have this counselling/therapy?			
Enter no. of treatments per month →			
OR if less than one per month			
Enter no. of treatments per year →			
Spontaneous: when needed......	1	1	1
(c) How long have you been having this counselling/therapy?			
Enter number of years →			
OR if less than 1 year			
Enter number of months → (less than 1 month = 0 0)			
(d) For what condition are you having this counselling/therapy? Obtain medical diagnosis AND describe main symptoms			
(e) Interviewer check: Is condition at B2(d) mentioned at B1(d), pages 4 and 5?	OFF USE	OFF USE	OFF USE
Yes.....	1→ col 2 or C1	1→ col 3 or C1	1 → C1
No.....	2→ (f)	2→ (f)	2→ (f)

Sched. B1C 8993 V4

10

Ring column number when appropriate →

	1	2	3
(f) DNA: Already asked about this condition in a previous column....	X	1 → col 3 or C1	1 → C1
Have you had any other treatment or medication for (CONDITION AT d) which you don't have now? Yes...... No......	1 → (g) / 2 → (i)	1 → (g) / 2 → (i)	1 → (g) / 2 → (i)
(g) Did you stop this treatment on your own accord or on professional advice? On own accord...... Professional advice......	1 → (h) / 2 → (i)	1 → (h) / 2 → (i)	1 → (h) / 2 → (i)
(h) What made you decide to stop this treatment? Code all that apply — Did not work/was not strong enough...... / Side effects...... / Other......	1 / 2 / 3	1 / 2 / 3	1 / 2 / 3
(i) Have you ever been offered any other treatment or medication for (CONDITION AT d) which you refused? Yes...... No......	1 → (j) / 2 → col 2 or C1	1 → (j) / 2 → col 3 or C1	1 → (j) / 2 → C1
(j) What was it?			
(k) Why did you refuse it? Code all that apply — Worry about side effects...... / Don't like medication/treatment...... / Other......	OFF USE 1 / 2 / 3	OFF USE 1 / 2 / 3	OFF USE 1 / 2 / 3

Sched. B1C 8993 V4

11

137

Blank page

C Health, social and voluntary care services

GP consultations

C1 During the two weeks ending yesterday, apart from any visit to a hospital, did you talk to a GP or family doctor on your own behalf, either in person or by telephone?

Yes .... 1 → (a)
No .... 2 → C2, page 14

(a) How many times have you talked to your GP or family doctor in the past two weeks?

Enter number of times → (b)

Ask (b) to (d) for the last 4 consultations (1 = most recent)

	1	2	3	4
Ring consultation number →				
(b) When you spoke to the doctor (on....occasion) did you talk about:				
a physical illness or complaint.	1	1	1	1
Running prompt or about being anxious or depressed, or a mental, nervous or emotional problem?	2	2	2	2
Spontaneous: Both of these	3	3	3	3
⊛ (c) Were you satisfied or dissatisfied with the consultation?				
Satisfied	1→col 2 or C2 / 2 → (d)	1→col 3 or C2 / 2 → (d)	1→col 4 or C2 / 2 → (d)	1 → C2 / 2 → (d)
Dissatisfied				
(d) In what way were you dissatisfied?				
Code all that apply Doctor does not listen, not interested, ignores me	1	1	1	1
Informant thinks treatment was inappropriate	2	2	2	2
Informant not given tests, treatment or hospitalisation	3	3	3	3
Doctor said there was nothing wrong or nothing s/he could do	4	4	4	4
Other	5	5	5	5

In patient stays

C2 During the past year, that is since (DATE) have you been in hospital as an in-patient, overnight or longer for treatment or tests?

[Include sight or hearing problems]

[Exclude giving birth]

Yes	1	→C3
No	2	→C5, page 16

C3 In the past 12 months, how many separate stays have you had in hospital as an in-patient?

Enter number of stays → ☐

C4 Ask (a) to (d) for the last 4 in-patient episodes (1=most recent)

Ring in-patient episode number →	1	2	3	4
(b) How many nights altogether were you in hospital on the (....) stay? Enter number of nights →	☐	☐	☐	☐

(c) Were you in hospital because of

	1	2	3	4
a physical health problem	1→col 2 or C5	1→col 3 or C5	1→col 4 or C5	1→C5
Running prompt or a mental nervous or emotional problem?	2 ⎤(c)	2 ⎤(c)	2 ⎤(c)	2 ⎤(c)
Spontaneous: Both	3 ⎦	3 ⎦	3 ⎦	3 ⎦

Schd. BLC 0393 V4

14

Ring in-patient episode number →	1	2	3	4
(e) Who referred you to hospital?				
GP	01	01	01	01
Community Psychiatric Nurse	02	02	02	02
Social worker	03	03	03	03
Psychiatrist	04	04	04	04
Via casualty (A and E)	05	05	05	05
Via law courts/Probation Service or Police	06	06	06	06
Self-admitted	07	07	07	07
Other	08	08	08	08
(d) When you were in hospital which people did you see? [Show card 15] [Exclude nurse with non specific duties] Code all that apply				
Psychiatrist/Psychotherapist	01	01	01	01
Other consultant or hospital doctor	02	02	02	02
Psychiatric Nurse	03	03	03	03
Social Worker/Counsellor	04	04	04	04
Occupational Therapist (OT)	05	05	05	05
Psychologist	06	06	06	06
Other	07	07	07	07

Schd. BLC 0393 V4

15

Out-patient episodes

C5 (Apart from seeing your own doctor/when you stayed in hospital) In the past 12 months have you been to a hospital or clinic or anywhere else for treatment or check-ups?

> Include visits to hospitals, day hospitals, clinics and private consulting rooms

Yes .... 1 → (a)
No .... 2 → C7, page 18

> Include attendance at day centres for treatment
> Exclude attendance at day centres for leisure
> Exclude sheltered workshops

(a) How many different places have you been for out-patient or day patient visits in the past year?

Enter number of places → [ ]

C6 For each place attended, ring column number and ask (a) to (f)

Ring column no.

	1	2	3	4
(a) Was your outpatient or day patient visit because of				
Running prompt a physical health problem	1→col 2 or C7	1→col 3 or C7	1→col 4 or C7	1→C7
or a mental, nervous or emotional problem?	2→(b)	2→(b)	2→(b)	2→(b)
Spontaneous - Both	3	3	3	3
(b) What type of place did you go to?				
Out-patient dept. of hospital	1	1	1	1
Casualty dept. of hospital	2	2	2	2
Clinic/Health Centre	3	3	3	3
Private consulting rooms	4	4	4	4
Day centre	5	5	5	5
Other	6	6	6	6
(c) How many times have you been to the (PLACE) in the past year? Enter no. of times. →	[ ]	[ ]	[ ]	[ ]

Sched. B LC 8X93 V4

Ring column no., when appropriate →

C6(d) Which of these people did you normally see at this hospital/clinic?

> Exclude nurse with non specific duties

[Show card 15]

	1	2	3	4
Code all that apply				
Psychiatrist/Psychotherapist	01	01	01	01
Other consultant/hospital doctor	02	02	02	02
Psychiatric Nurse	03	03	03	03
Social worker/Counsellor	04	04	04	04
Occupational Therapist (OT)	05	05	05	05
Psychologist	06	06	06	06
Other	07	07	07	07
(e) Are you currently attending (PLACE)? Yes	1→col 2 or C7	1→col 3 or C7	1→col 4 or C7	1→C7
No	2→(f)	2→(f)	2→(f)	2→(f)
(f) Have you stopped going on your own accord or were you discharged? On own accord	1	1	1	1
Discharged	2	2	2	2

Sched. B LC 8X93 V4

C7 Here is a list of people who visit people in their homes to give
them help and support when they need it.
Have any of these people visited you in the past year?

Yes...... 1 →(a)
No ...... 2 →C8, page 20

Show card 16

Ring person no.
Code all that apply →

	Community Psychiatric Nurse	Occupational Therapist	Social Worker	Psychiatrist	Home care worker/ Home help	Voluntary Worker	Second Voluntary Worker
	1	2	3	4	5	6	7

(a) How often does (PERSON) come?

Show card 17

	Community Psychiatric Nurse	Occupational Therapist	Social Worker	Psychiatrist	Home care worker/ Home help	Voluntary Worker	Second Voluntary Worker
4 or more times a week	1	1	1	1	1	1	1
2 or 3 times a week	2	2	2	2	2	2	2
Once a week	3	3	3	3	3	3	3
Less often than once a week but at least once a month	4	4	4	4	4	4	4
Less often than once a month	5	5	5	5	5	5	5

b) How satisfied or dissatisfied are you with the help or support (PERSON) gives you? Are you

Running prompt *

	Community Psychiatric Nurse	Occupational Therapist	Social Worker	Psychiatrist	Home care worker/ Home help	Voluntary Worker	Second Voluntary Worker
very satisfied	1	1	1	1	1	1	1
fairly satisfied	2	2	2	2	2	2	2
fairly dissatisfied	3	3	3	3	3	3	3
or very dissatisfied?	4	4	4	4	4	4	4

c) Ask for voluntary worker(s) if applicable
Which voluntary organisation does (PERSON) come from?

	Voluntary Worker	Second Voluntary Worker
Voluntary worker does not come from any organisation	1	1
MIND	2	2
Manic Depression Fellowship	3	3
Phobic Action/Society	4	4
National Schizophrenia Fellowship	5	5
Cruse	6	6
Alcohol concern	7	7
Standing conference on Drug Abuse	8	8
Other	9	9

18

19

Sched. BLC 0393 V4

141

C8 [Show card 18]

In the past year, have you been offered any help or support from any of the people listed on this card, or indeed any other service, **which you turned down?**

Yes	1 → (a)
No	2 → C9

(a) What sort of help/service were you offered?

Code all that apply

Community Psychiatric Nurse	1
Occupational Therapist/Industrial Therapist	2
Social Worker/Counselling Service	3
Psychiatrist	4
Home care worker/Home help	5
Voluntary Worker	6
Other	7

[*] **(b)** Did you turn it down because you did not want or need the help or for some other reason?

Code all that apply

Did not want/need help	1
Could not face it/handle it	2
Did not like people/not the right people offering help	3
Didn't think it could/would help	4
Inconvenient time or location	5
Other reason	6

C9 Sometimes people do not see a doctor or other professional about mental, nervous or emotional problems when perhaps they should. In the past year did you decide not to see a doctor or other professional when either you or people around you thought you should?

Yes	1 → (a)
No	2 → Section D

[*] **(a)** Thinking about the last time this happened, what were your reasons for not going to a doctor or other professional?

Write verbatim and then code

Code all that apply

Didn't know who to go to or where to go	01
Did not think anyone could help	02
Hour inconvenient/didn't have the time	03
Thought problem would get better by itself	04
Too embarrassed to discuss it with anyone	05
Afraid what family/friends would think	06
Family or friends objected	07
Afraid of consequences (treatment, tests, hospitalisation, sectioned)	08
Afraid of side effects of any treatment	09
Didn't think it was necessary/ No problem	10
A problem one should be able to cope with	11
Other	12

→ Section D

D. Practical activities

[*]

Do you have any difficulty . . . . .

	(a) Do you need anyone to help you (. . . . .)?	Yes	No	DNA		(c) Who helps you . .	Code all that apply from list	Yes	No
D1	With personal care such as dressing, bathing, washing, or using the toilet?	with personal care?	1	2	3	with personal care?	□ □ □ □	1	2
D2	Getting out and about or using transport?	getting out and about?	1	2	3	getting out and about	□ □ □ □	1	2
D3	With medical care such as taking medicines or pills, having injections or changes of dressing?	with medical care?	1	2	3	with medical care?	□ □ □ □	1	2
D4	With household activities like preparing meals, shopping, laundry and housework?	with household activities?	1	2	3	with household activities?	□ □ □ □	1	2
D5	With practical activities such as gardening, decorating, or doing household repairs?	with practical activities?	1	2	3	with practical activities?	□ □ □ □	1	2
D6	Dealing with paperwork, such as writing letters, sending cards or filling in forms?	dealing with paperwork?	1	2	3	dealing with paperwork?	□ □ □ □	1	2
D7	Managing money, such as budgeting for food or paying bills?	managing money?	1	2	3	managing money?	□ □ □ □	1	2

List

00	No one
01	Spouse/cohabitee
02	Brother/sister (incl. in-law)
03	Son/daughter (incl. in-law)
04	Parent (incl. in-law)
05	Grandparent (incl. in-law)
06	Grandchild (incl. in-law)
07	Other relative
08	Boyfriend/girlfriend
09	Friend
10	CPN/Nurse
11	Occupational Therapist
12	Social worker
13	Home care worker/home help
14	Voluntary worker
15	Landlord/landlady
16	Paid domestic help
17	Paid nurse
18	Bank manager
19	Solicitor
20	Other person

A - N1361B Mar93 V4

22   23

Recent Life Events   DNA: Proxy interviews................ [1] → **Go to Section E, page 28**

The following questions are about events or problems which may have happened to you during the past 6 months which might have caused you distress and to seek help

Use **card 19** if subject not alone, otherwise, ask D8 to D13

Then ask **(a)** to **(g)** if coded 1 at main

		(a) When did this happen? More than 6 months = 6 Less than 1 month = 0	(b) Was there anyone, among your family or friends, who understood what this felt like?		(c) And were you able to talk about it openly and get support and understanding?	
	Yes | No	No of months since event	Yes	No	Yes	No
D8 In the past 6 months, have you yourself suffered from a serious illness, injury or an assault?	1 | 2	☐	1 → (c)	2 → (d)	1	2
D9 (In the past 6 months,) has a serious illness, injury or an assault happened to a close relative?	1 | 2	☐	1 → (c)	2 → (d)	1	2
D10 (In the past 6 months,) has a parent, spouse (or partner), child, brother or sister of yours died?	1 | 2	☐	1 → (c)	2 → (d)	1	2
D11 (In the past 6 months,) has a close family friend or another relative died, such as an aunt, cousin or grandparent?	1 | 2	☐	1 → (c)	2 → (d)	1	2
D12 (In the past 6 months,) have you had a separation due to marital difficulties or broken off a steady relationship?	1 | 2	☐	1 → (c)	2 → (d)	1	2
D13 (In the past 6 months,) have you had a serious problem with a close friend, neighbour or relative?	1 | 2	☐	1 → (c)	2 → (d)	1	2

(d) Did you get any professional help, for this, that is from someone other than family or friends?		(e) Did you try to get help for this, from any professional?		(f) Was this because you didn't know where to get the help you wanted from or because you felt you didn't need any professional help?			(g) Was it help with practical things or did you need someone to talk things over with?		
Yes	No	Yes	No	DK where	Didn't need help		Practical	Talk over	Both
1 → (g)	2 → (e)	1 → (g)	2 → (f)	1 → (g)	2 → See D9		1	2 → See D9	3
1 → (g)	2 → (e)	1 → (g)	2 → (f)	1 → (g)	2 → See D10		1	2 → See D10	3
1 → (g)	2 → (e)	1 → (g)	2 → (f)	1 → (g)	2 → See D11		1	2 → See D11	3
1 → (g)	2 → (e)	1 → (g)	2 → (f)	1 → (g)	2 → See D12		1	2 → See D12	3
1 → (g)	2 → (e)	1 → (g)	2 → (f)	1 → (g)	2 → See D13		1	2 → See D13	3
1 → (g)	2 → (e)	1 → (g)	2 → (f)	1 → (g)	2 → Go to D14		1	2 → Go to D14	3

Now I'd like to ask you about some other events or problems which may have happened to you during the past 5 months.

Use card 20 if subject not alone, otherwise, ask D14 to D18

Then ask (a) to (g) if coded 1 at main

D14 In the past 6 months, were you made redundant or sacked from your job?

D15 (In the past 6 months,) were you seeking work without success for more than one month?

D16 (In the past 6 months,) did you have a major financial crisis, such as losing the equivalent of 3 months income?

D17 (In the past 6 months,) did you have problems with the police involving a court appearance?

D18 (In the past 6 months,) was something you valued lost or stolen?

	Yes / No	(a) When did this happen? No of months since event	(b) Was there anyone among your family or friends, who understood what this felt like? Yes / No	(c) And were you able to talk about it openly and get support and understanding? Yes / No
D14	1 2	□	1 → (c) 2 → (d)	1 2
D15	1 2	□	1 → (c) 2 → (d)	1 2
D16	1 2	□	1 → (c) 2 → (d)	1 2
D17	1 2	□	1 → (c) 2 → (d)	1 2
D18	1 2	□	1 → (c) 2 → (d)	1 2

More than 6 months = 6
Less than 1 month = 0

A N161B Mar93 V4

(d) Did you get any professional help for this, that is from someone other than family or friends? Yes / No	(e) Did you try to get help for this, from any professional? Yes / No	(f) Was this because you didn't know where to get the help you wanted from or because you felt you didn't need any professional help? DK where / Didn't need help	(g) Was it help with practical things or did you need for someone to talk things over with? Practical / Talk over / Both
1 → (g) 2 → (e)	1 → (g) 2 → (f)	1 → (g) 2 → See D15	1 2 3 See D15
1 → (g) 2 → (e)	1 → (g) 2 → (f)	1 → (g) 2 → See D16	1 2 3 See D16
1 → (g) 2 → (e)	1 → (g) 2 → (f)	1 → (g) 2 → See D17	1 2 3 See D17
1 → (g) 2 → (e)	1 → (g) 2 → (f)	1 → (g) 2 → See D18	1 2 3 See D18
1 → (g) 2 → (e)	1 → (g) 2 → (f)	1 → (g) 2 → Go to Section E	1 2 3 Go to Section E

A N161B Mar93 V4

E Social Life

E1. The next few questions are about how you spend your leisure time.

When you are at home, what sorts of things do you usually do during your leisure time?

Show card 21

Code all that apply

		(a)	
		Share	Do on own
Entertaining friends or relatives	01		
Writing letters/telephoning	02		
Reading books and newspapers	03		
TV/radio	04	1	2
Listening to music	05	1	2
Hobbies inc. art and crafts, knitting, playing a musical instrument, writing poetry	06	1	2
Gardening	07	1	2
DIY/ car maintenance	08	1	2
Games inc. cards, computer games, betting and gambling	09	1	2
Other leisure pursuits	10	1	2
Spontaneous: No leisure time/no leisure pursuits	99		→ Go to E3

(a) **Ask for each activity informant does except for 'entertaining friends or relatives', 'writing letters/telephoning' and 'reading books and newspapers':**

Refer to activity and ask:

Is this an interest which you share with someone else and usually do together or do you usually do it on your own?

Ring code in column (a) above. Then go to E2.

E2. What sorts of things do you usually do during your leisure time away from home?

Show card 22

Code all that apply

		(a)	
		Share	Do on own
Visiting friends or relatives	01		
Pubs, restaurants	02	1	2
Night clubs, discos	03	1	2
Clubs, organisations	04	1	2
Classes, lectures	05	1	2
Going for a walk, walking the dog	06	1	2
Sports inc. keep fit, cycling, swimming, football and horse riding	07	1	2
Sports as a spectator	08	1	2
Cinema, theatre, concerts	09	1	2
Bingo, amusement arcades	10	1	2
Bookmakers, betting and gambling	11	1	2
Shopping	12	1	2
Church	13	1	2
Political activities	14	1	2
Library	15	1	2
Other leisure pursuits	16	1	2
Spontaneous: No leisure time/no leisure pursuits	99		→ Go to E3

(a) **Ask for each activity informant does except for 'entertaining friends or relatives':**

Refer to activity and ask:

Is this an interest which you share with someone else and usually do/go to together or do you usually do it/go on your own?

Ring code in column (a) above.

E3. Do you go to any of these places for social activities?

		Yes	No
(a)	Day centre?	1	2
(b)	Club for people with physical health problems?	1	2
(c)	Club for people with mental health problems?	1	2
(d)	Any other types of social club?	1	2

Individual prompt

E4. Do you regularly go to . . . . .

(a)	an Adult Education Centre?	1	2
(b)	an Adult Training Centre?	1	2

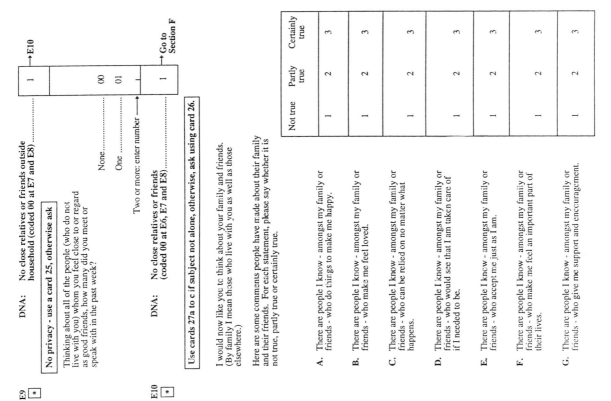

E9. *

DNA: No close relatives or friends outside household (coded 00 at E7 and E8) .... 1 → E10

No privacy - use a card 25, otherwise ask

Thinking about all of the people (who do not live with you) whom you feel close to or regard as good friends, how many did you meet or speak with in the past week?

None 00
One 01
Two or more: enter number → 1 → Go to Section F

E10. *

DNA: No close relatives or friends (coded 00 at E6, E7 and E8) .... 1 → Go to Section F

Use cards 27a to c if subject not alone, otherwise ask using card 26.

I would now like you to think about your family and friends. (By family I mean those who live with you as well as those elsewhere.)

Here are some comments people have made about their family and their friends. For each statement, please say whether it is not true, partly true or certainly true.

	Not true	Partly true	Certainly true
A. There are people I know - amongst my family or friends - who do things to make me happy.	1	2	3
B. There are people I know - amongst my family or friends - who make me feel loved.	1	2	3
C. There are people I know - amongst my family or friends - who can be relied on no matter what happens.	1	2	3
D. There are people I know - amongst my family or friends - who would see that I am taken care of if I needed to be.	1	2	3
E. There are people I know - amongst my family or friends - who accept me just as I am.	1	2	3
F. There are people I know - amongst my family or friends - who make me feel an important part of their lives.	1	2	3
G. There are people I know - amongst my family or friends - who give me support and encouragement.	1	2	3

31

A-N1361 Mar93 V2

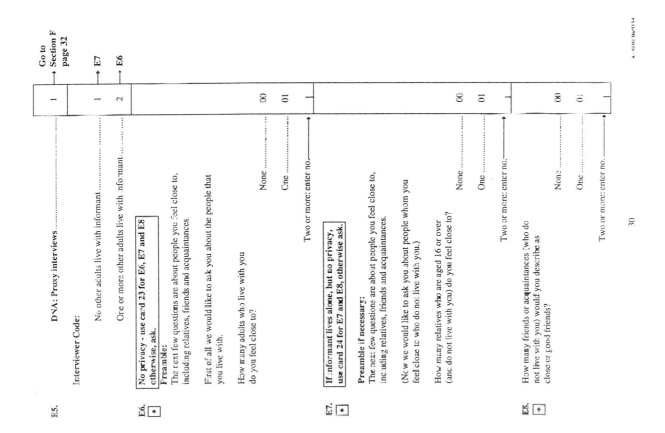

E5.

DNA: Proxy interviews .... 1 → Go to Section F page 32

Interviewer Code:
No other adults live with informant .... 1 → E7
One or more other adults live with informant .... 2 → E6

E6. *

No privacy - use card 23 for E6, E7 and E8 otherwise, ask.

Preamble:
The next few questions are about people you feel close to, including relatives, friends and acquaintances.

First of all we would like to ask you about the people that you live with.

How many adults who live with you do you feel close to?

None 00
One 01
Two or more: enter no →

E7. *

If informant lives alone, but no privacy, use card 24 for E7 and E8, otherwise ask.

Preamble if necessary:
The next few questions are about people you feel close to, including relatives, friends and acquaintances.

(Now we would like to ask you about people whom you feel close to who do not live with you.)

How many relatives who are aged 16 or over (and do not live with you) do you feel close to?

None 00
One 01
Two or more: enter no →

E8. *

How many friends or acquaintances (who do not live with you) would you describe as close or good friends?

None 00
One 01
Two or more: enter no →

30

A-N1361 Mar93 V4

F   Education and Employment Status

F1.   At what age did you finish your continuous full-time education at school or college?

Not yet finished	1
Never went to school	2
14 or under	3
15	4
16	5
17	6
18	7
19 or over	8

32

F2.   Please look at this card and tell me whether you have passed any of the qualifications listed. Look down the list and tell me the first one you come to that you have passed.

Show card 28

Degree (or degree level qualification)	1
Teaching qualification HNC/HND, BEC/TEC Higher, BTEC Higher City and Guilds Full Technological Certificate	2
Nursing qualifications (SRN, SCM, RGN, RM RHV, Midwife	
'A' levels/SCE higher ONC/OND/BEC/TEC **not** higher City and Guilds Advanced/Final level	3
'O' level passes (Grade A - C if after 1975) GCSE (Grades A - C) CSE Grade 1 SCE Ordinary (Bands A - C) Standard Grade (Level 1 - 3) SLC Lower SUPE Lower or Ordinary School Certificate or Matric. City and Guilds Craft/Ordinary level	4
CSE Grades 2 - 5 GCE 'O' level (Grades D & E if after 1975) GCSE (Grades D, E, F, G) SCE Ordinary (Bands D & E) Standard Grade (Level 4, 5) Clerical or commercial qualifications Apprenticeship	5
CSE ungraded	6
Other qualifications (specify)	7
No qualifications	8

Code first that applies

33

A - N361 B M4v93 V4

A - N361 B M4

F5. Interviewer check

Had a job last week (coded 01 at F3 or 02 at F3(a))	1	→ **F8**
Unemployed waiting to take up a job (coded 03 at F3(a)(i))	2	→ **F6**
Unemployed looking for work (coded 04 or 05 at F3(a)(i))	3	→ **F7**
Others - economically inactive (coded 06 to 10 at F3(a)(i))	4	→ **F7**

F6. Unemployed waiting to take up a job

Apart from the job you are waiting to take up, have you ever had a paid job or done any paid work?

Yes	1	→ **F8**
No	2	

F7. All others unemployed and economically inactive

(May I check) have you ever had a paid job or done any paid work?

Yes	1	→ **F8**
No	2	→ **See F20, page 41**

35

Employment status

F3. Did you do any paid work in the last week, that is in the 7 days ending last Sunday, either as an employee or self employed?

Yes	01	→ **F5**
No	02	→ (a)

> **Include paid sheltered employment**
> **Include work based training schemes**
> **Exclude college based training schemes**

(a) Even though you weren't working, did you have a job that you were away from last week?

Yes	02	→ **F4**
No		→ (i)

(i) Last week were you:

Code first applies

waiting to take up a job that you had already obtained?	03	
looking for work?	04	
intending to look for work but prevented by **temporary** ill-health, sickness or injury?	05	
going to school or college full time? **(use only for persons aged 16 - 49)**	06	
permanently unable to work because of long term sickness or disability? **(for women, use only if aged 16 - 59)**	07	
retired? **(use only if stopped work at age 50 or over)**	08	
looking after the home or family?	09	
or were you doing something else?	10	→ **F5**

F4. What was the **main** reason you were away from work (last week)?

Code one only

On leave/holiday	1	
A mental, nervous or emotional problem	2	
A physical health problem	3	
Attending a training course away from the workplace	4	
Laid off/short time	5	
Personal/family reason	6	
Other reasons	7	→ **F5**

34

F8. If employed
(i) What was your job last week?

If not employed
(ii) What was your most recent job?

(iii) What is the job you are waiting to take up?

If retired
(iv) What was your main job?

Job title:

Description:

Industry:

SOC

IND

(a) **Informant's Definition**
Full-time 1
Part-time 2

(b) Employee .... 1 → F9
Self-employed .... 2 → F10

F9 (a) If employee ask or record
Manager 1
Foreman/supervisor ... 2
other employee 3

(b) How many employees work(ed) in the establishment
1 - 24 1
25 - 499 2
500 or more ... 3

(c) Do/did you work in sheltered employment such as with:

Running Prompt
Remploy 1
a local authority 2
a blind association 3
a voluntary association 4
or in a sheltered place with an ordinary employer? 5
DK/None of these 6

F10 If self employed
Do/did you employ other people?
Yes, PROBE: 1 - 24 1
25 - 499 2
500 or more ... 3
No employees 4

F11. To those with a job last week (coded 1 at F5, page 35)

DNA: Unemployed/Economically Inactive .... 1 → See F18, page 40

A. For employees (main job/government scheme)
How long have you been with your present employer (up to yesterday)?

B. For self-employed (main job)
How long have you been self-employed (up to yesterday)?

Show Card 29 and prompt as necessary

Less than 4 weeks 01
4 weeks but less than 3 months 02
3 months but less than 6 months 03
6 months but less than 12 months 04
12 months but less than 2 years 05
2 years but less than 3 years 06
3 years but less than 5 years 07
5 years but less than 10 years 08
10 years but less than 15 years 09
15 years but less than 20 years 10
20 years but less than 25 years 11
25 years but less than 30 years 12
30 years but less than 35 years 13
35 years but less than 40 years 14
40 years or more 15

F12. A. For employees (main job/government scheme)
(introduce if on short time/lay-off:
I'd like to ask about your hours when you are not on short time/laid off ...)

How many hours a week do you usually work (in your main job/government scheme), that is **excluding meal breaks and overtime?**

NO OF HOURS excluding meal breaks and overtime

Check with informant that this is excluding any paid or unpaid overtime

B. For self-employed, (main job)
(Introduce if on short time/lay-off:
I'd like to ask about your hours when you are not on short time/laid off ...)

How many hours a week in total do you usually work (in your main job), that is **excluding meal breaks but including any overtime**

TOTAL HOURS excluding meal breaks

Check with informant that this is total hours including any paid or unpaid overtime

If work pattern not based on a week, give average over a few months

F14. To those with a job last week but temporarily not working because of a mental or physical health problem (coded 2 or 3 at F4, page 34)

DNA: Others .... 1 → See F26, page 43

How long have you been off work?

Less than 2 weeks	1	
2 weeks, less than 1 month	2	
1 month, less than 3 months	3	
3 months, less than 6 months	4	
6 months or more	5	

F15. If employee   DNA: Self-employed (coded 2 at F8(b), page 36) .... 4 → **F16**

[*] Do you expect to return to your present employer?

Yes .... 1 → (a)
No .... 2 → **F16**
Not sure 3

(a)   Do you expect to return to the same job?

Yes .... 1 → See F26, page 43
No 2
DK 3

F16. Do you expect to be fit to work again?

[*] Yes .... 1 → **F17**
No .... 2 → See F26, page 43
Not sure 3

F17. Will you look for another paid job in the future?

[*] Yes .... 1 → See F26, page 43
No .... 2 → (a)
DK 3

(a) Why will/may you not look for another job?

[*] **Code all that apply**

No suitable jobs: general employment situation .... 1 → See F26, page 43
No suitable jobs: due to health problems 2
Too old 3
Other 4

F13.

DNA: Proxy interview .... 1 → See F26, page 43

[*] Earlier I was asking you about how you had been feeling in the past month.

Has your health or the way you have been feeling caused you to take time off work in the past year?

Yes .... 1 → (a)
No .... 2 → **F14**

(a) How many days in the past year have you taken off work?

Enter number of days →

Weekends falling within a period of sickness must be included

F18. If not working but has worked

DNA: Never worked (coded 2 at F6, page 35) ...... 1 → See F20

How old were you when you left your last paid job?

Enter age ____ → See F26, page 43

F19. DNA: Proxy interview ...... 1 → See F26, page 43

[*] Did a mental, nervous or emotional problem have anything to do with your leaving your last job?

Yes ...... 1 → (a)

No ...... 2 → See F20

(a) DNA: Self-employed in last job (coded 2 at F8 (b) page 36) ...... 1 → See F20

Did your employer ask you to leave or did you leave of your own accord?

Employer asked ...... 1 → See F20

Left of own accord 2

40

F20. DNA: Proxy interview ...... 1 → See F26, page 43

DNA: Retired (code 08 at F3(a)(i), page 34) ...... 1 → See F26, page 43

If not working but not retired

[*] Is the reason that you are not working at present that ...

Code first that applies

the way you have been feeling makes it impossible for you to do any kind of paid work? ...... 1 → (a)

a physical health problem makes it impossible for you to do any kind of paid work? ...... 2 → F21

you have not found a suitable paid job? ...... 3 → F21

or because you do not want or need a paid job? ...... 4 → See F26, page 43

Other ...... 5 → F21

[*] (a) May I just check, would you be able to do some kind of sheltered or part-time work if it were available, or is this impossible?

Could do sheltered work ...... 1 → F21

Could do part-time work 2

Impossible to do work ...... 3 → See F26, page 43

F21. (May I just check) Are you looking for a job at the moment?

[*] Yes ...... 1 → F23

No ...... 2 → (a)

[*] (a) Have you looked for a job at all (since you last worked)?

Yes ...... 1 → F22

No ...... 2 → (i)

[*] (i) Why have you not looked for a job?

Code all that apply

No suitable jobs around - general employment situation ...... 1 → See F26, page 43

No suitable jobs for someone with subject's health problem 2

Other 3

F22. Why have you stopped looking for jobs?

[*] Code all that apply

No suitable jobs around - general employment situation 1

No suitable jobs for someone with subject's health problem 2

Other 3

41

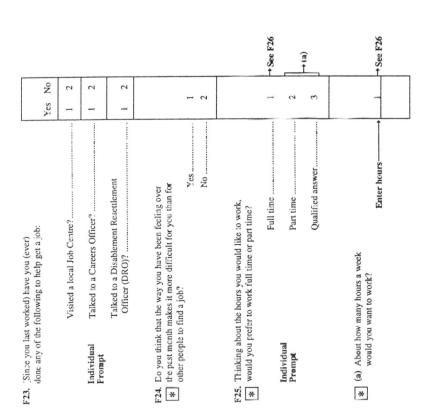

F23. Since you last worked) have you (ever)
done any of the following to help get a job:

	Yes	No
Visited a local Job Centre?	1	2
Talked to a Careers Officer?	1	2
Talked to a Disablement Resettlement Officer (DRO)?	1	2

Individual Prompt

F24. Do you think that the way you have been feeling over
the past month makes it more difficult for you than for
other people to find a job?

* Yes 1
No .... 2 → See F26

F25. Thinking about the hours you would like to work,
would you prefer to work full time or part time?

*
Full time 1
Individual Prompt
Part time .... 2 → (a)
Qualified answer .... 3 → See F26

* (a) About how many hours a week
would you want to work?
Enter hours ⟶

A-N1361 B Mar93 V4

42

F26. Spouse's employment

DNA: no spouse .... 1 → Section G, p 45

Enter person no. of spouse
(from H'hold box) ⟶

I'd now like to ask you about (SPOUSE).

Did (SPOUSE) do any paid work in the last week,
that is in the 7 days ending last Sunday,
either as an employee or self-employed?

Yes .... 01 → F27
No .... ⌐ → (a)

(a) Even though he/she wasn't working, did he/she
have a job that he/she was away from last week?

Yes .... 02 → F27
No .... ⌐ → (i)

(i) Last week was he/she:

Code first that applies

waiting to take up a job that he/she
had already obtained? 03

looking for work? 04

intending to look for work but
prevented by temporary sickness
or injury? 05

going to school or college full time?
(use only for persons aged 16 - 49) .... 06 → (ii)

permanently unable to work because of
long term sickness or disability?
(for women, use only if aged 16 - 59) 07

retired?
(use only if stopped work at aged 50 or over) 08

looking after the home or family? 09

or was he/she doing something else? 10

(ii) May I check, has he/she ever had a paid job
or done any paid work?

Yes .... 1 → F27
No .... 2 → Section G, p 45

A-N1361 B Mar93 V4

43

153

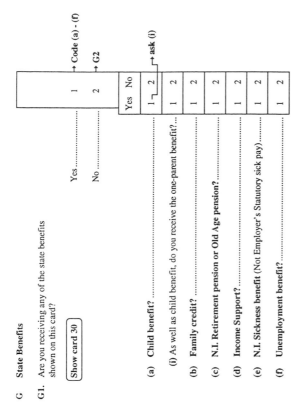

G   State Benefits

G1. Are you receiving any of the state benefits shown on this card?

Show card 30

Yes .... 1 → Code (a) - (f)

No .... 2 → G2

	Yes	No
(a) Child benefit?	1	2 → ask (i)
(i) As well as child benefit, do you receive the one-parent benefit?	1	2
(b) Family credit?	1	2
(c) N.I. Retirement pension or Old Age pension?	1	2
(d) Income Support?	1	2
(e) N.I. Sickness benefit (Not Employer's Statutory sick pay)	1	2
(f) Unemployment benefit?	1	2

45

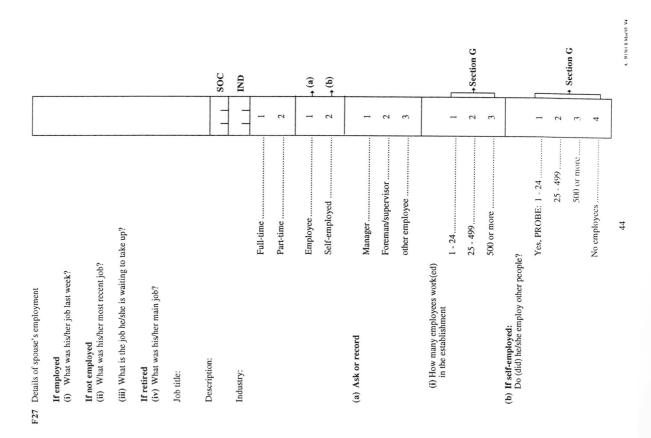

F27   Details of spouse's employment

If employed
(i)   What was his/her job last week?

If not employed
(ii) What was his/her most recent job?

(iii) What is the job he/she is waiting to take up?

If retired
(iv) What was his/her main job?

Job title:

Description: SOC

Industry: IND

Full-time 1

Part-time 2

Employee .... 1 → (a)

Self-employed .... 2 → (b)

(a) Ask or record

Manager 1

Foreman/supervisor ... 2

other employee 3

(i) How many employees work(ed) in the establishment

1 - 24 1

25 - 499 .... 2 → Section G

500 or more 3

(b) If self-employed:
Do (did) he/she employ other people?

Yes, PROBE: 1 - 24 ... 1

25 - 499 2

500 or more .... 3 → Section G

No employees 4

44

Other Income

G3. (In addition to these), do you receive income from any of the sources on this card?

> Show card 32

Yes ..... 1 → Code (a) - (f)
No ..... 2 → G4

	Yes	No
(a) **Earned Income/salary?**	1	2
(b) **Income from self-employment?**	1	2
(c) **Pension from a former employer?**	1	2
(d) **Interest from savings, building society, investment dividends from shares etc?**	1	2
(e) **Other kinds of regular allowances from outside the household (eg alimony, annuity, educational grant)?**	1	2
(f) Any other source?(specify)	1	2

G4. Could you please look at this card and tell me which group represents your own personal gross income from all sources mentioned?

By gross income, I mean income from all sources before deductions for income tax and National Insurance.

> Show card 33

(a) Enter group number ————→
  or
  DK 98
  Refused ..... 99 → See section H page 49

(a) **Ask, or if single person household, record group no. at G4**

Could you look at the card again and tell me which group represents your household's gross income from all sources.

> Show card 33

Enter group number ————→
  or
  DK 98
  Refused 99

G2. (In addition) are you receiving any of the State benefits listed on this card or any other N.I. or State benefit (for example, war benefits or maternity allowance)?

> Show card 31

Yes ..... 1 → Code (a) - (m)
No ..... 2 → G3

	Yes	No
(a) **Widow's pension or War Widow's pension?**	1	2
(b) **Any other State Widow's benefit (eg Widowed Mother's allowance)?** [Exclude Widow's benefit]	1	2
(c) **War disablement pension?**	1	2
(d) **Invalidity pension, Invalidity benefit or allowance?**	1	2
(e) **Severe disablement allowance?**	1	2
(f) **Mobility allowance?**	1	2
(g) **Industrial disablement allowance?**	1	2
(h) **Attendance allowance?**	1	2
(i) **Disability Living allowance?**	1	2
(j) **Disability Working allowance?**	1	2
(k) **Invalid care allowance?**	1	2
(l) **Maternity allowance?**	1	2
(m) **Anything else? (Specify)**	1	2

155

H **Smoking**

H1 Have you ever smoked a cigarette, a cigar, or a pipe?

DNA: Proxy interview	1 → Complete front page
Yes	1 → H2
No	2 → Go to Section I, page 52

H2. Do you smoke cigarettes at all nowadays?

Yes	1 → H3
No	2 → H10

H3. About how many cigarettes a **day** do you usually smoke at weekends?

Less than 1	00
No. smoked a day	⌐

H4. And about how many cigarettes a **day** do you usually smoke on weekdays?

Less than 1	00
No. smoked a day	⌐

H5. Do you mainly smoke

Running prompt
Code one only

filter-tipped cigarettes	1 ⌐ → H6
or plain or untipped cigarettes	2
or hand-rolled cigarettes?	3 → H7

H6. Which brand of cigarette do you usually smoke?

Enter details	Full brand name	
	Size e.g. King, luxury, regular	
	Filter tipped or plain	

INTERVIEWER: Code from reference card C

Not on list.........	1 → H7

Blank page

H7. How easy or difficult would you find it to go without smoking for a whole day?

Running prompt

Very easy......	1
Fairly easy......	2
Fairly difficult......	3
Very difficult?......	4
DK......	5

H8. Would you like to give up smoking altogether?

Yes......	1
No......	2
DK......	3

H9. How soon after waking do you **usually** smoke your first cigarette of the day?

Less than 5 minutes......	1
5 - 14 minutes......	2
15 - 29 minutes......	3
30 minutes but less than 1 hour......	4
1 hour but less than 2 hours......	5
2 hours or more......	6 → **H11**

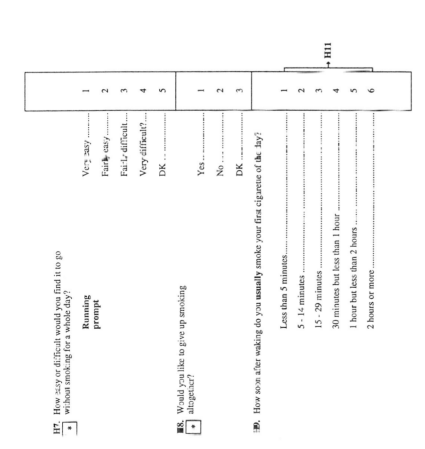

50

A. N136 B Mar93 V4

H10. Have you ever smoked cigarettes regularly?

Yes......	1 → **(a)**
No......	2 → **H12**

(a) About how many cigarettes did you smoke in a day when you smoked them regularly?

Less than 1	00

No. smoked a day

(b) How long ago did you stop smoking cigarettes regularly?

Less than 6 months ago......	1
6 months but less than a year ago......	2
1 year but less than 2 years ago......	3
2 years but less than 5 years ago......	4
5 years but less than 10 years ago......	5
10 years or more ago......	6 → **H11**

H11. How old were you when you started to smoke cigarettes regularly?

Enter age →	
Spontaneous: Never smoked cigarettes regularly	00 → **H12**

H12. Do you smoke at least one cigar of any kind per month nowadays?

Yes......	1 → **(a)**
No......	2 → **(b)**

(a) About how many cigars do you usually smoke in a week?

Less than 1	00 → **See H13**

No. smoked a week

(b) Have you ever regularly smoked at least one cigar of any kind per month?

Yes......	1 → **See H13**
No......	2 → **See H13**

H13. To all men who have ever smoked (Coded 1 at H1)

DNA: Women	1 → **Go to Section I page 52**

Do you smoke a pipe at all nowadays?

Yes......	1 → **Go to Section I page 52**
No......	2 → **H14**

H14. Have you ever smoked a pipe regularly?

Yes......	1 → **Go to Section I page 52**
No......	2	

51

A. N136 B Mar93 V4

157

I Drinking

I1. I'm now going to ask you a few questions about what you drink - that is, if you do drink.

Do you ever drink alcohol nowadays, including drinks you brew or make at home?

Yes	1	→I5
No	2	→I2

I2. Could I just check, does that mean you never have an alcoholic drink nowadays, or do you have an alcoholic drink very occasionally, perhaps for medicinal purposes or on special occasions like Christmas or New Year?

Very occasionally	1	→I5
Never	2	→I3

I3. Have you always been a non-drinker, or did you stop drinking for some reason?

Always a non-drinker	1	→I4(a)
Used to drink but stopped	2	→I4(b)

I4(a). Always a non drinker

[*] Why is that?

Code all that apply

Religious reasons	1	
Don't like it	2	
Parent's advice	3	Go to self completion, page 6, then complete front page
Health reasons	4	
Can't afford it	5	
Other	6	

I4(b). Used to drink but stopped

[*] What would you say was the main reason you stopped drinking?

Code all that apply

Religious reasons	1	
Don't like it	2	
Parent's advice	3	Go to self completion, page 6, then complete front page
Health reasons	4	
Can't afford it	5	
Other	6	

A. NIMB Mar93 V4

I5. I'm going to read out a few descriptions about the amounts of alcohol people drink, and I'd like you to say which one fits you best.
[*] Would you say you:

Running prompt

hardly drink at all	1	
drink a little	2	
drink a moderate amount	3	→I6
drink quite a lot	4	
or drink heavily?	5	
DK	6	

A. NIMB Mar93 V4

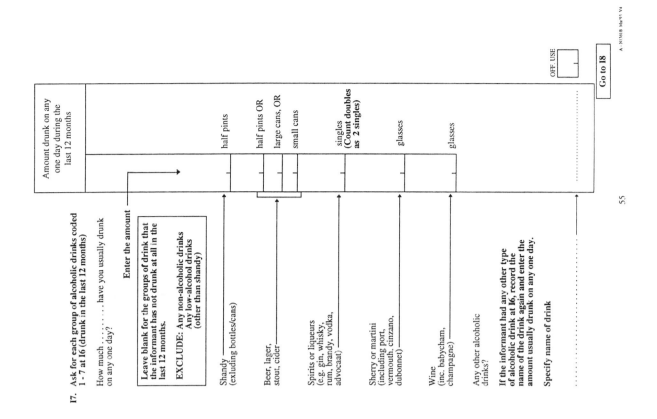

I7. Ask for each group of alcoholic drinks coded 1 - 7 at I6 (drunk in the last 12 months)

How much . . . . have you usually drunk on any one day?

Enter the amount

Leave blank for the groups of drink that the informant has not drunk at all in the last 12 months.

EXCLUDE: Any non-alcoholic drinks
Any low-alcohol drinks (other than shandy)

Amount drunk on any one day during the last 12 months

Shandy (excluding bottles/cans) — half pints

Beer, lager, stout, cider — half pints OR / large cans, OR / small cans

Spirits or liqueurs (e.g. gin, whisky, rum, brandy, vodka, advocaat) — singles **(Count doubles as 2 singles)**

Sherry or martini (including port, vermouth, cinzano, dubonnet) — glasses

Wine (inc. babycham, champagne) — glasses

Any other alcoholic drinks?

If the informant had any other type of alcoholic drink at I6, record the name of the drink again and enter the amount usually drunk on any one day.

Specify name of drink

OFF. USE

Go to I8

A - N1361B Mar93 V4

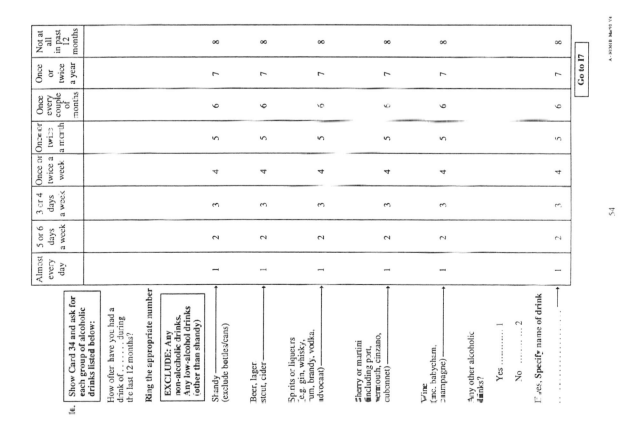

I6. Show Card 34 and ask for each group of alcoholic drinks listed below:

How often have you had a drink of . . . . during the last 12 months?

Ring the appropriate number

EXCLUDE: Any non-alcoholic drinks. Any low-alcohol drinks (other than shandy)

	Almost every day	5 or 6 days a week	3 or 4 days a week	Once or twice a week	Once or twice a month	Once every couple of months	Once or twice a year	Not at all in past 12 months
Shandy (exclude bottles/cans)	1	2	3	4	5	6	7	8
Beer, lager stout, cider	1	2	3	4	5	6	7	8
Spirits or liqueurs (e.g. gin, whisky, rum, brandy, vodka, advocaat)	1	2	3	4	5	6	7	8
Sherry or martini (including port, vermouth, cinzano, dubonnet)	1	2	3	4	5	6	7	8
Wine (inc. babycham, champagne)	1	2	3	4	5	6	7	8
Any other alcoholic drinks?	1	2	3	4	5	6	7	8

Yes 1
No 2

If yes, Specify name of drink . . . .

Go to I7

A - N1361B Mar93 V4

I8. During the past year, how often did you have 12 or more **units** of alcoholic drink of any kind in a single day, that is any combination of beers, glasses of wine, or other alcoholic drinks?

This card will help you to work out the number of units.

Show card 34 and use cards 35 and 36 as necessary

Almost every day .... 1 → Go to page 2 of self completion, then complete front page

5 - 6 days a week 2

3 - 4 days a week 3

Once or twice a week 4

Once or twice a month 5

Once or twice in 6 months 6

Once or twice a year .... 7 → I9

Not at all in the past 12 months 8

I9. During the past year, how often did you have from 8 to 11 **units** of alcoholic drink of any kind in a single day, that is any combination of beers, glasses of wine, or other alcoholic drinks?

Show card 34 and use cards 35 and 36 as necessary

Almost every day .... 1 → Go to page 2 of self completion, then complete front page

5 - 6 days a week 2

3 - 4 days a week 3

Once or twice a week 4

Once or twice a month 5

Once or twice in 6 months 6

Once or twice a year .... 7 → I9

Not at all in the past 12 months 8

A - N136B Mar/93 V4

I10. During the past year, how often did you have from 5 to 7 **units** of alcoholic drink of any kind in a single day, (that is any combination of beers, glasses of wine, or other alcoholic drinks)?

Show card 34 and use cards 35 and 36 as necessary

Almost every day 1

5 - 6 days a week .... 2 → Go to page 2 of self completion, then complete front page

3 - 4 days a week 3

Once or twice a week 4

Once or twice a month 5

Once or twice in 6 months .... 6 → Go to page 6 of self completion, then complete front page

Once or twice a year 7

Not at all in the past 12 months 8

A - N136B Mar/93 V4

D

N1361

Self-Completion

IN CONFIDENCE

Stick serial number label

H'hld

Date of interview

| | | 9 | 3 |

Part A

Here is a list of some experiences that many people have reported in connection with drinking.

Please read each item and indicate if this has ever happened to you in the past 12 months.

	Please ring 1 or 2 for each item	
	Yes	No
1. I have skipped a number of regular meals while drinking	1	2
2. I have often had an alcoholic drink the first thing when I got up in the morning	1	2
3. I have had a strong drink in the morning to get over the effects of the previous night's drinking	1	2
4. I have woken up the next day not being able to remember some of the things I had done while drinking	1	2
5. My hands shook a lot the morning after drinking	1	2
6. I need more alcohol than I used to, to get the same effect as before	1	2
7. My drinking has interfered with my spare time activities or hobbies	1	2
8. Sometimes I have needed a drink so badly that I couldn't think of anything else	1	2
9. Sometimes I have woken up during the night or early morning sweating all over because of drinking	1	2
10. I have got into a heated argument while drinking	1	2
11. I have got into a fight in a pub while drinking	1	2
12. I have got into a fight at home while drinking	1	2
13. A police officer questioned or warned me because of my drinking	1	2

	Please ring 1 or 2 for each item	
	Yes	No
14. My drinking contributed to getting involved in an accident in which someone else was hurt or property, such as a car, was damaged	1	2
15. My drinking contributed to my getting hurt in an accident in a car or elsewhere	1	2
16. I had trouble with the police about drinking when driving was not involved	1	2
17. I have been arrested for driving after drinking	1	2
18. I have stayed drunk for several days at a time	1	2
19. Once I started drinking it was difficult for me to stop before I became completely drunk	1	2
20. I sometimes kept on drinking after I promised myself not to	1	2
21. I deliberately tried to cut down or stop drinking, but I was unable to do so	1	2
22. I had an illness connected with drinking which kept me from working or doing my regular activities for a week or more	1	2
23. I felt that my drinking was becoming a serious threat to my physical health	1	2
24. A doctor suggested that I cut down on my drinking	1	2
25. I have lost a job or nearly lost one because of drinking	1	2

Now, please turn over

Blank page

26. In the past 12 months, did any of the people in the list below, ask you to drink less or to act differently when you were drinking?

Yes .... 1 → **Go to (a)**

No .... 2 → **Please turn to page 6**

1.	Spouse or partner
2.	Mother
3.	Father
4.	Girlfriend or boyfriend
5.	Any other relative
6.	Anyone else you live with
7.	Any other friend
8.	Someone else

(a) Who asked you to drink less or act differently when you were drinking? Please circle number(s) in the box below.

For example, if your mother and father asked you to drink less, circle '2' and '3' below.

1	2	3	4	5	6	7	8

→ **Go to (b)**

(b) Did this threaten or break up your relationship with any of the people who asked you to drink less or act differently?

Yes .... 1 → **Go to (c)**

No .... 2 → **Now please turn to page 6**

(c) Which relationship(s) did this threaten or break up? Please circle number(s) in the box below.

1	2	3	4	5	6	7	8

→ **Now please turn to page 6**

Part B

Now I'd like to ask about your experience with drugs.
Here is a list of the most commonly used drugs.

1. Sleeping Pills, Barbiturates, Sedatives, Downers, Seconal
2. Tranquillisers, Valium, Librium
3. Cannabis, Marijuana, Hash, Dope, Grass, Ganja, Kif
4. Amphetamines, Speed, Uppers, Stimulants, Qat
5. Cocaine, Coke, Crack
6. Heroin, Smack
7. Opiates other than heroin: Demerol, Morphine, Methadone, Darvon, Opium, DF118
8. Psychedelics, Hallucinogens: LSD, Mescaline, Acid, Peyote, Psylocybin (Magic)mushrooms
9. Ecstasy
0. Solvents, inhalants, glue, amyl nitrate

Please look at the above list and answer questions A, B and C

A Have you _ever_ used any of the drugs on the list more than was prescribed for you?

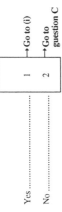

Yes .... 1 → Go to (i)
No .... 2 → Go to question B

(i) Which of these drugs have you used more than was prescribed for you?
Please circle the category/categories of drugs from the list in the box below.

1 2 3 4 5 6 7 8 9 0 → Go to question B

Now please answer question B on the opposite page.

B Have you _ever_ used any of the drugs on the list to get high?

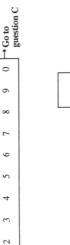

Yes .... 1 → Go to (i)
No .... 2 → Go to question C

(i) Which of these drugs have you used to get high?
Please circle the category/catergories of drugs from the list in the box below.

1 2 3 4 5 6 7 8 9 0 → Go to question C

C Have you _ever_ used any of the drugs on the list without a prescription?

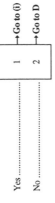

Yes .... 1 → Go to (i)
No .... 2 → Go to D

(i) Which of these drugs have you used without a prescription?
Please circle the category/categories of drugs from the list in the box below.

1 2 3 4 5 6 7 8 9 0 → Go to D

D **If you have answered 'yes' to any of questions A, B or C, please go to question 1 on the next page.**

If you have answered 'no' to all of questions A, B and C, please hand this back to the inteviewer.

164

1.	Sleeping Pills, Barbiturates, Sedatives, Downers, Seconal
2.	Tranquillisers, Valium, Librium
3.	Cannabis, Marijuana, Hash, Dope, Grass, Ganja, Kif
4.	Amphetamines, Speed, Uppers, Stimulants, Qat
5.	Cocaine, Coke, Crack
6.	Heroin, Smack
7.	Opiates other than heroin: Demerol, Morphine, Methadone, Darvon, Opium, DF118
8.	Psychedelics, Hallucinogens: LSD, Mescaline, Acid, Peyote, Psylocybin (Magic mushrooms)
9.	Ecstasy
0.	Solvents, inhalants, glue, amyl nitrate

Please answer the following questions thinking about the drugs on this list which you have used without a prescription, to get high, or more than was prescribed for you.

1. Have you *ever* used any of the drugs more than five times in your life?

Yes .... 1 → Go to (a)
No .... 2 → Go to Q15, page14

(a) What was it? (What are they?)
Please circle the category/categories of drugs from the list.

1 2 3 4 5 6 7 8 9 0 → Go to (b)

(b) In what year did you first use any of the drugs on this list?

Please enter year — 19 [ ] → Go to 2

2. Have you used any one of these drugs in the past 12 months?

Yes .... 1 → Go to (a)
No .... 2 → Go to Q15, page 14

(a) What was it? (What were they?)
Please circle category/categories of drugs from the list.

1 2 3 4 5 6 7 8 9 0 → Go to Q3

3. Have you ever used any one of these drugs every day for two weeks or more in the past 12 months?

Yes .... 1 → Go to (a)
No .... 2 → Go to Q4

(a) What was it? (What were they?)
Please circle category/categories of drugs from the list.

1 2 3 4 5 6 7 8 9 0 → Go to Q4

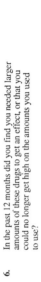

1. Sleeping Pills, Barbiturates, Sedatives, Downers, Seconal
2. Tranquillisers, Valium, Librium
3. Cannabis, Marijuana, Hash, Dope, Grass, Ganja, Kif
4. Amphetamines, Speed, Uppers, Stimulants, Qat
5. Cocaine, Coke. Crack
6. Heroin, Smack
7. Opiates other than heroin: Demerol, Morphine, Methadone, Darvon, Opium, DF118
8. Psychedelics, Hallucinogens: LSD, Mescaline, Acid, Peyote, Psylocybin (Magic)mushrooms
9. Ecstasy
0. Solvents, inhalants, glue, amyl nitrate

4. In the past 12 months have you used any one of these drugs to the extent that you felt like you needed it or were dependent on it?

Yes .... 1 → Go to (a)
No .... 2 → Go to Q5

(a) What was it? (What were they?)
Please circle category/categories of drugs from the list.

1 2 3 4 5 6 7 8 9 0 → Go to Q5

5. In the past 12 months have you tried to cut down on any drugs but found you couldn't do it?

Yes .... 1 → Go to (a)
No .... 2 → Go to Q6

(a) What was it? (What were they?)
Please circle category/categories of drugs from the list.

1 2 3 4 5 6 7 8 9 0 → Go to Q6

N345 SC D.I.C 0393 V2

6. In the past 12 months did you find you needed larger amounts of these drugs to get an effect, or that you could no longer get high on the amounts you used to use?

Yes .... 1 → Go to (a)
No .... 2 → Go to Q7

(a) What was it? (What were they?)
Please circle category/categories of drugs from the list.

1 2 3 4 5 6 7 8 9 0 → Go to Q7

7. In the past 12 months, have you had withdrawal symptoms, such as feeling sick because you stopped or cut down on any of these drugs?

Yes .... 1 → Go to (a)
No .... 2 → Go to Q8

(a) What was it? (What were they?)
Please circle category/categories of drugs from the list.

1 2 3 4 5 6 7 8 9 0 → Go to Q8

8. In the past 12 months did you have any health problems, such as fits, an accidental overdose, a persistent cough or an infection as a result of using any of these drugs?

Yes .... 1 → Go to (a)
No .... 2 → Go to Q9

(a) What was it? (What were they?)
Please circle category/categories of drugs from the list.

1 2 3 4 5 6 7 8 9 0 → Go to Q9

N345 SC D.I.C 0393 V2

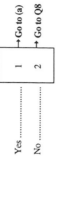

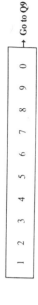
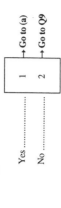
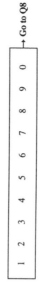
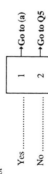

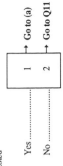

1. Sleeping Pills, Barbiturates, Sedatives, Downers, Seconal

2. Tranquillisers, Valium, Librium

3. Cannabis, Marijuana, Hash, Dope, Grass, Ganja, Kif

4. Amphetamines, Speed, Uppers, Stimulants, Qat

5. Cocaine, Coke, Crack

6. Heroin, Smack

7. Opiates other than heroin: Demerol, Morphine, Methadone, Darvon, Opium, DF118

8. Psychedelics, Hallucinogens: LSD, Mescaline, Acid, Peyote, Psylocybin (Magic mushrooms)

9. Ecstasy

0. Solvents, inhalants glue, amyl nitrate

9. In the past 12 months did any drugs cause you considerable problems with your family or friends, at work or at school or with the police?

Yes .... 1 → Go to (a)
No .... 2 → Go to Q10

(a) What drug was it? (What were they?) Please circle category/categories of drugs from the list.

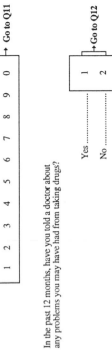

1 2 3 4 5 6 7 8 9 0 → Go to Q10

12

---

10. In the past 12 months did you have any emotional or psychological problems from taking drugs, such as feeling crazy or paranoid, or depressed or uninterested in things?

Yes .... 1 → Go to (a)
No .... 2 → Go to Q11

(a) What drug was it? (What were they?) Please circle category/categories of drugs from the list.

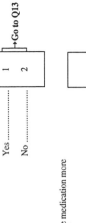

1 2 3 4 5 6 7 8 9 0 → Go to Q11

11. In the past 12 months, have you told a doctor about any problems you may have had from taking drugs?

Yes .... 1 → Go to Q12
No 2

12. In the past 12 months, have you spoken to any other professional about any problems you may have had from taking drugs?

Yes .... 1 → Go to Q13
No 2

13. In the past 12 months, did you use medication more than once for any drug problems?

Yes .... 1 → Go to Q14
No 2

14. In the past 12 months, did you have any drug problems which interfered with your life or activities a lot?

Yes .... 1 → Go to Q15, page 14
No 2

13

168

15. May I just check, have you ever injected yourself with drugs?

Yes .... 1 → Go to (a)

No .... 2 → **Thank you for filling this in. Please hand it back to the interviewer.**

(a) Have you ever shared injection equipment with someone else?

Yes 1

No .... 2 → **Go to Q16**

16. Have you injected a drug in the past month?

Yes .... 1 → Go to (a)

No .... 2 → **Thank you for filling this in. Please hand it back to the interviewer.**

(a) Have you shared injection equipment with someone else in the past month?

Yes 1

No 2

Thank you for filling this in. Please hand it back to the interviewer.

Appendix D: Statistical terms and their interpretation

D.1 Comorbidity

Odds ratios were used in the assessment of the degree of comorbidity between the disorders. Here, the term comorbidity is used to refer to the co-occurrence of two psychiatric disorders. This association between disorders can be expressed in terms of an odds ratio: that is, how much the presence of one disorder increased the odds of having a second. For example, Table 6.22 shows that depression and phobia were strongly associated: a diagnosis of the former increased the odds of having the latter disorder more than 11-fold. The confidence interval does not include 1.00, indicating that the association between these two disorders was unlikely to be due to chance.

D.2 Confidence intervals

The means and percentages quoted in the text of this report represent summary information about a variable (e.g., CIS-R score) based on the sample of people interviewed in this study. However, extrapolation from these sample statistics is required in order to make inferences about the distribution of that particular variable in the population. This is done by calculating confidence intervals around the statistic in question. These confidence intervals indicate the range within which the 'true' (or population) percentage is likely to lie. Where 95% confidence intervals are calculated, this simply indicates that one is '95% confident' that the population percentage lies within this range. (More accurately, it indicates that if repeated samples were drawn from the population, the true percentage would lie within this range in 95% of the samples.)

Confidence intervals are calculated on the basis of the sampling error (q.v.). The upper 95% confidence intervals are calculated by adding the sampling error multiplied by 1.96 to the sample percentage or mean. The lower confidence interval is derived by subtracting the same value. 99% confidence intervals can also be calculated, by replacing the value 1.96 by the value 2.58.

D. 3 Multiple logistic regression (MLR) and Odds Ratios

(i) Interpretation of odds ratios

Chapters four to six of this report use logistic regression analysis to provide a measure of the effect of various socio-demographic variables on psychiatric symptoms, on CIS-R scores and on disorders. Unlike many of the cross-tabulations presented elsewhere in the report, MLR estimates the effect of any socio-demographic variable while controlling for the confounding effect of other variables in the analysis. A forward stepwise method of logistic regression was used. The dependent variable was dichotomous, indicating the presence or absence of a particular symptom or disorder. All the socio-demographic variables were categorical.

Logistic regression produces an estimate of the odds of a symptom/disorder being present when an individual is in a particular category of a socio-demographic variable compared to a reference category of that variable. The odds of having a disorder are defined as the ratio of the probability of the disorder being present compared with the probability of the disorder not being present. If the probability of having a disorder is p, the odds are $p/(1-p)$. The factor by which the odds of a disorder differ for people in a particular category compared with those in the reference category is shown by the Adjusted Odds Ratio (OR). The OR controls for the possible confounding effects of the other variables in the statistical model, e.g. age, employment status, family unit type and locality. For example, Table 6.14 shows adults categorised into family unit type 'lone parent & child(ren)' were almost three times more likely to have a depressive episode compared with those in the reference category of 'couple, no children' (adjusted odds ratio = 2.60). To determine whether the increased odds of having a disorder are due to chance rather than having a particular characteristic, one must consult the confidence interval associated with the odds ratio (see ii).

Asterisks in the tables presenting odds ratios in this Report indicate that within a particular characteristic, differences in odds between the reference group and the other group(s) were significant. For example, in Table 6.14 the OR associated with being in the category 'lone parent with child(ren)' is marked with an asterisk to show a significant increase in odds of having a depressive episode compared with those in the reference group, 'couple, no child(ren)'. However, the tables do not indicate significant differences between two non-reference groups, for example, within family unit type, a significant difference between the categories 'lone parent & child(ren)' and 'couple & child(ren)' would not be marked. Also, significant differences between categories across characteristics are not marked; a significant difference between people in the category 'couple, no child(ren)' with those categorised as 'unemployed' would not be marked. In some tables there are characteristics where no significant relationships were found between the reference group and other groups, i.e. none of the non-reference groups are marked with an asterisk. The fact that these characteristics were nevertheless selected by the model means that significant relationships must exist between two or more of the non-reference groups.

Selection of reference groups

a) Dichotomous variables, for example male/female and manual/non-manual: in these cases it made no difference which was selected as the reference group.

b) Ordinal variables ordered from one extreme to another, e.g. age, qualifications: one end of the range was selected as the reference group.

c) Nominal variables with more than two groupings where the categories had no logical order, for example family unit type and ethnicity: the group with the lowest prevalence of 'any neurotic disorder' was selected as the reference group.

(ii) Confidence intervals around an Odds Ratio

The confidence intervals around odds ratios can be interpreted in the manner described earlier in this section. For example, Table 6.14 shows an odds ratio of 2.60 for the category 'lone parent with child(ren)' with a confidence interval ranging from 1.60 to 4.26, indicating that the 'true' (i.e., population) OR is 95%

likely to lie between these two values. If the confidence interval does not include 1.00 then the OR is likely to be significantly different from that of the reference category.

D.4 Sampling errors

The sampling error is a measure of the degree to which a percentage (or other summary statistic) would vary if repeatedly calculated in a series of samples. For example, if the mean CIS-R score was calculated in a random sample of men drawn from the population at large, then another sample was drawn and the mean calculated again, its value would be unlikely to be identical to the first mean. If this process was continued, the sample mean would continue to vary from sample to sample. The sampling error provides a measure of this variability among sample means, and is used in the calculation of confidence intervals and statistical significance tests. In this survey simple random sampling did not take place; rather, multi-stage stratified sampling was used. Sampling errors were therefore calculated using an in-house software package (EPSILON) specifically written to calculate sampling errors for this design of survey. This does not affect the interpretation of the sampling errors or their use in the calculation of confidence intervals.

D.5 Significance

It is stated in the text of the Report that some differences and some odds ratios are 'significant'. This indicates that it is unlikely that an odds ratio of this magnitude would be found due to chance alone. Specifically, the likelihood that the OR shows an effect simply by chance is less than 5%. This is conventionally assumed to be infrequent enough to discount chance as an explanation for the finding.

Glossary of survey definitions and terms

Adults
In this survey adults were defined as persons aged 16 or over and less than aged 65.

Antipsychotic drugs
These are also known as 'neuroleptics'. In the short term they are used to quieten disturbed patients whatever the underlying psychopathology.
See Depot Injections

Depot injections
When antipsychotic medication is given by injections on a monthly basis, these are sometimes termed depot injections.

Educational level
Educational level was based on the highest educational qualification obtained and was grouped as follows:

Degree (or degree level qualification)

Teaching, HND, Nursing
    Teaching qualification
    HNC/HND, BEC/TEC Higher, BTEC Higher
    City and Guilds Full Technological Certificate
    Nursing qualifications:
    (SRN,SCM,RGN,RM,RHV,
    Midwife)

A level
    GCE A-levels/SCE higher
    ONC/OND/BEC/TEC/not higher
    City and Guilds Advanced/Final level
O level
    GCE O-level (grades A-C if after 1975)
    GCSE (grades A-C)
    CSE (grade 1)
    SCE Ordinary (bands A-C)
    Standard grade (levels 1-3)
    SLC Lower SUPE Lower or Ordinary
    School certificate or Matric
    City and Guilds Craft/Ordinary level

GCSE/CSE
    GCE O-level (grades D-E if after 1975)
    GCSE (grades D-G)
    CSE (grades 2-5)
    SCE Ordinary (bands D-E)
    Standard grade (levels 4-5)

    Clerical or commercial qualifications
    Apprenticeship
    Other qualifications

No qualifications
    CSE ungraded
    No qualifications

Employment Status
Four types of employment status were identified: working full time, working part time, unemployed and economically inactive.

Working adults
The two categories of working adults include persons who did any work for pay or profit in the week ending the last Sunday prior to interview, even if it was for as little as one hour, including Saturday jobs and casual work (e.g. babysitting, running a mail order club).

Self-employed persons were considered to be working if they worked in their own business, professional practice, or farm for the purpose of making a profit, or even if the enterprise was failing to make a profit or just being set up.

The unpaid 'family worker' (e.g., a wife doing her husband's accounts or helping with the farm or business) was included as working if the work contributed directly to a business, farm or family practice owned or operated by a related member of the same household. (Although the individual concerned may have received no pay or profit, her contribution to the business profit counted as paid work.) This only applied when the business was owned or operated by a member of the same household.

Anyone on a Government scheme which was employer based was also 'working last week'.

Informants' definitions dictated whether they felt they were working full time or part time.

Unemployed adults
This category included those who were waiting to take up a job that had already been obtained, those who were looking for work, and people who intended to look for work but were prevented by

temporary ill-health, sickness or injury. 'Temporary' was defined by the informant.

Economically inactive
This category comprised five main categories of people:

'Going to school or college' only applied to people who were under 50 years of age. The category included people following full-time educational courses at school or at further education establishments (colleges, university, etc). It included all school children (16 years and over).

During vacations, students were treated as 'going to school or college' even where their return to college was dependent on passing a set of exams. If however, they were having a break from full-time education, i.e. they were taking a year out, they were not counted as being in full-time education.

'Permanently unable to work because of long-term sickness or disability' only applied to those under state retirement age, ie to men aged 16 to 64 and to women aged 16 to 59. 'Permanently' and 'long-term' were defined by the informant.

'Retired' only applied to those who retired from their full-time occupation at age 50 or over and were not seeking further employment of any kind.

'Looking after the home or family' covered anyone who was mainly involved in domestic duties, provided this person had not already been coded in an earlier category.

'Doing something else' included anyone for whom the earlier categories were inappropriate.

Ethnicity
Household members were classified into nine groups by the person answering Schedule A.

White	White
Black - Caribbean	
Black - African	West Indian/African
Black - Other	
Indian	
Pakistani	
Bangladeshi	Asian/Oriental
Chinese	
None of these	Other

For analysis purpose these nine groups were

subsumed under 4 headings: White, West Indian/African, Asian/Oriental and Other.

Family unit
In order to classify the relationships of the subject to other members of the households, the household members were divided into family units.

Subjects were assigned to a family unit depending on whether they were or ever had been married, and whether they (or their partners) had any children living with them.

A 'child' was defined for family unit purposes as an adult who lives with one or two parents, provided he or she has never been married and has no child of his or her own in the household.

For example, a household containing three women, a grandmother, mother and child would contain two family units with the mother and child being in one unit, and the grandmother being in another. Hence family units can consist of:

- A married or cohabiting couple or a lone parent with their children

- Other married or cohabiting couples

- An adult who has previously been married. If the adult is now living with parents, the parents are treated as being in a separate family unit

- An adult who does not live with either a spouse, partner, child or parent. This can include adults who live with siblings or with other unrelated people, e.g. flatmates.

Family unit type
Each informant's family unit was classified into one of six family unit types:

'Couple no children' included a married or cohabiting couple without children.

'Couple with child' comprised a married or cohabiting couple with at least one child from their liaison or any previous relationship.

'Lone parent' describes both men and women (who may be single, widowed, divorced or separated) living with at least one child. The subject in this case could be a divorced man looking after his 12 year-old son or a 55 year-old widow looking after a 35 year-old, daughter who had never married and had no children of her own.

'One person' describes the family unit type and does not necessarily mean living alone. It includes people living alone but includes one person living with a sister, or the grandmother who is living with her daughter and her family. It also includes adults living with unrelated people in shared houses, e.g. flatmates.

'Adult living with parents' describes a family unit which has the same members as 'couple with child' but in this case it is the adult son or daughter who is the subject. It includes a 20 year old unmarried student living at home with married or cohabiting parents, and a 62 year old single woman caring for her elderly parents.

'Adult living with lone parent' covers the same situations as above except that there is one and not two parents in the household.

Household

The standard definition used in most surveys carried out by OPCS Social Survey Division, and comparable with the 1991 Census definition of a household, was used in this survey. A household is defined as a single person or group of people who have the accommodation as their only or main residence and who either share one meal a day or share the living accommodation. (See E McCrossan *A Handbook for interviewers*. HMSO: London 1985.)

Locality

Interviewers coded their opinion of whether the sampled address was in an urban, semi-rural or rural area.

Marital status

Informants were categorised according to their own perception of marital status. Married and cohabiting took priority over other categories. Cohabiting included anyone living together with their partner as a couple.

Psychiatric morbidity

The expression psychiatric morbidity refers to the degree or extent of the prevalence of mental health problems within a defined area.

Region

When the survey was carried out there were 14 Regional Health authorities in England. These were the basis for stratified sampling and have been retained for purposes of analysis. Scotland and Wales were treated as two distinct areas.

Social class

Based on the Registrar General's 1991 *Standard Occupational Classification,* Volume 3 OPCS, HMSO: London social class was ascribed on the basis of the following priorities:

Firstly, social class was based on the informant's own occupation, unless the informant was a married or cohabiting woman. In such cases, the spouse or partner's occupation was used. The exception is where the spouse or partner had never worked, in which case the woman's own occupation was used.

Secondly, social class was based on the informant' (or spouse's) current occupation or, if the informant (or spouse) was unemployed or economically inactive at the time of interview but had previously worked, social class was based on the most recent previous occupation.

The classification used in the tables is as follows:

Descriptive definition	Social class
Professional	I
Intermediate occupations	II
Skilled occupations — non-manual	III NM
Skilled occupations — manual	III M
Partly-skilled	IV
Unskilled occupations	V
Armed Forces	

Social class was not determined where the subject (and spouse) had never worked, or if the subject was a full-time student or where occupation was inadequately described.

Tenure

Four tenure categories were created:

'Owned outright' means bought without mortgage or loan or with a mortgage or loan which has been paid off.

'Owned with mortgage' includes co-ownership and shared ownership schemes.

'Rent from LA/HA' means rented from local authorities, New Town corporations or commissions or Scottish Homes, and housing associations which include co-operatives and property owned by charitable trusts.

'Rent from other source' includes rent from organisations (property company, employer or other organisation) and from individuals (relative, friend, employer or other individual).

Type of accommodation

Four types of accommodation were created:

'Detached' means a detached house or bungalow.

'Semi-detached' includes a semi-detached whole house or bungalow.

'Terraced' means a terraced or end of terraced whole house or bungalow.

'Flat/maisonette' includes a purpose built flat or maisonette in block, converted flat or maisonette in a house, a room in a house or block, a bedsit.

Printed in the United Kingdom for HMSO.
Dd.0300612, 4/95, C25, 3400, 5673, 322608.